EAT FOR HEALTH

A Do-It-Yourself Nutrition Guide
for Solving Common Medical Problems

William D. Manahan, M.D.

H J Kramer Inc
Tiburon, California

Published by H J Kramer Inc
P.O. Box 1082
Tiburon, CA 94920

ISBN 0-915811-11-1
Library of Congress Catalog Card Number: 88-81722

Editor: Suzanne Lipsett
Cover art: Genevieve Wilson
Cover design: Jon Tedesco
Typesetter: TBH Typecast, Inc.
Editorial Assistant: Nancy Carleton
Book production: Schuettge & Carleton

Manufactured in the United States of America

10   9   8   7   6   5   4   3   2   1

Foreword

Dr. William Manahan wrote *Eat for Health* to help "empower *you* to improve *your own* health." The clear steps he outlines will enable you to solve many common medical problems on your own. But this is not just another self-help book; it is the result of years of passionate effort on the part of its author to help people achieve better health. Nutrition counseling has played a major role in Dr. Manahan's large and successful medical practice. Over the years, Dr. Manahan has seen many of his patients' lives improve dramatically through simple dietary changes. With the information Dr. Manahan provides in this book, you, too, can take positive steps to improve your diet and your health.

Chapters dealing with caffeine, salt, sugar, fats, milk, and processed foods pinpoint specific problem areas and give the reader a better understanding of the relationships between food, health, and disease. Throughout this book, Dr. Manahan helps you identify the elements in your diet that are causing you problems. The chapters on milk and dairy products may seem revolutionary to some readers; the concept that dairy sensitivity is related to a wide range of health problems is still not universally accepted. Dr. Manahan does an excellent job in clarifying this relationship.

The best of information is of little use without an action plan. The most significant contribution of this book is that it emphasizes implementation; it shows you how to take concrete action based on your new knowledge of nutrition and of the problems caused by certain foods. Dr. Manahan takes a "non-faddish" approach toward healthful eating habits. Drawing upon the current recommendations of the American Heart Association, the National Cancer Institute, and the dietary goals of federal health agencies, he gives the reader authentic tools for developing a healthier life-style.

I extend my congratulations to Dr. Manahan for his excellent contribution to all of us concerned about health improvement and a healthy diet for everyone, from kids through seniors. This book will have an important place not only in the library but in the kitchens of all concerned readers.

Jeffrey Bland, Ph.D.
Gig Harbor, Washington
May 31, 1988

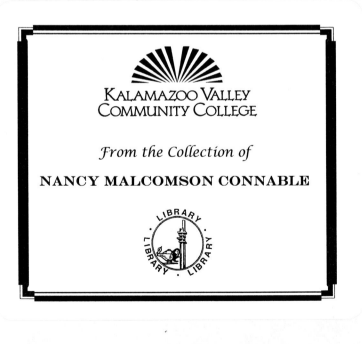

Acknowledgments

Many people have helped and encouraged me during the writing of *Eat for Health*. There are a special few on whom I wish to bestow extra kudos.

Herrick Peterson, former editor of *Patient Care*, generously helped with the initial rewrites.

Marty Heiberg at *Postgraduate Medicine* was most helpful with her editing.

Special thanks go to librarian Ruth Ann Engstrom. She cheerfully and tirelessly obtained hundreds of articles and books for me.

Barb Hanson and her word processor were invaluable. I also learned that every writer needs his or her own word processor!

Linda Hachfeld, the dietician at our Wellness Center, did a wonderful job of helping me examine both sides of many controversial dietary issues. I'm especially grateful to Linda and to my brother, Jim Manahan, for proofreading the book.

My wonderful sons, Michael, David, Tim, and Topher, deserve a special martyr's award for tolerating their father's changing and unending quest for a more healthy diet.

Working with my publishers, Hal and Linda Kramer, has been a wonderful experience. They have been sensitive and receptive to my needs and wants. Thank you, Hal and Linda.

For inspiration, my thanks go to five different people. Diane Manahan, my best friend, colleague, and wife, and Chuck Lofy, my friend and colleague, have continually encouraged me to dream the impossible dream and to keep on tilting at windmills. The other three people who inspired me are the nutritional gurus from whom I have learned so much: Jeff Bland, John McDougall, and Jonathon Wright.

My final thanks go to the two groups of wonderful people to whom I wish to dedicate this book. Both groups have been vital forces in keeping me on the winding path of continued learning. These two sensational groups of people are the members of the American Holistic Medical Association and all of my patients. To the people belonging to these two groups, I must say thank you and I love you all!

William D. Manahan

Contents

Preface

Welcome! Writing this book has been a labor of love for me. During the course of my active family practice over the past sixteen years, I have become more and more excited about my discovery that many of my patients' problems have simple dietary solutions. Often, merely eliminating a single food from the diet alleviates a symptom or cures a disease that has been troubling a person for months or even years.

For example, you can imagine the excitement both John, a patient, and I felt, when his intermittent headaches of three years' duration suddenly vanished, never to return again, after he quit drinking coffee. Robert, another patient, was both angry and happy when he discovered that the three or four glasses of milk he was drinking each day to help his duodenal ulcer were actually making it worse. Robert's heartburn, abdominal pain, and stomach gurgling went away completely following a two-week dairy-elimination diet. His anger and frustration were directed at me because I had not told him that milk increases acid output in the stomach and might actually be harmful to some people with ulcers.

Now, you may wonder why I, as Robert's physician, had not told him about this side effect of milk. The reason was simply that I had not known about it. In fact, until recently, no physician knew this fact—or knew, for that matter, that caffeine frequently causes headaches.

Over the past decade, more and more findings of this kind have been uncovered. Therefore, practicing medicine has grown increasingly exciting for me over the same time period. Many people to whom I could offer no solutions previously are now able to eliminate or ease serious and debilitating symptoms by making nutritional changes. For me, that is exciting and rewarding!

Despite tremendous nutritional discoveries made over the past decade, physicians in general have remained both uninterested and uninformed about the subject. Why that is, I'm not sure. But I do know, after a decade of speaking to groups of people about nutrition, that most patients are interested in the subject. Many realize that accurate nutritional knowledge can help them eliminate serious, painful, or debilitating health problems. People outside the medical establishment are "hungry" for nutritional information and its relationship to disease.

I wrote this book to empower *you* to improve *your own* health — to help you inform yourself of the relationship between how you feel and what you eat. It will enable you to discover ways of getting rid of many of your symptoms. You may even find out how to prevent some diseases that run in your family and that have been of concern to you for years.

The symptoms and diseases hypothesized or proven to be related to food intake are listed in the index. Simply look up the one you are concerned about, read the information pertinent to that problem, and then decide if you want to try the recommended dietary changes. Robert, the man mentioned above, could have looked up ulcers, heartburn, or abdominal pain. The index would have directed him to those pages containing information on milk, caffeine, and artificial sweeteners. Since Robert was neither a user of artificial sweeteners nor a coffee drinker but was a four-cup-per-day milk drinker, it would have been up to him to decide if he wanted to go on the suggested fourteen-day milk-elimination trial diet to determine whether milk was affecting his stomach. Robert's abdominal pains and heartburn would have improved significantly with the elimination diet. He would have achieved this improvement without seeing a physician and without spending a cent.

This book presents simple, fast, inexpensive ways of reducing symptoms and eliminating many diseases without professional assistance. Does it sound too easy? Too unsophisticated? Try it! You'll be amazed, just as John and Robert were. It still astounds me that all these different symptoms and diseases could possibly be related to what we eat or drink. Of course, nutrition is just *one* of the multiple causes of most problems, but it is an area that we have tended to overlook.

You can play a part by sending me your own nutritional solutions. If *your* solution is published in a revised edition, you will be given credit for it. So let me hear from you!

William D. Manahan, M.D.
124 Ridgely Road
Mankato, Minnesota 56001

Introduction

What "Eating Well" Really Means

Is the way you feel linked to what you eat? If you feel less than great a good part of the time, that's a question worth looking into. And if you have a significant health problem or fear that you might have one, it's a question you can't afford to ignore. The aim of this book is to give you a simple, personal answer to this important question. It will start you on a course that could lead to a powerful feeling of worry-free well-being.

This book identifies six culprits in the modern diet that cause the largest numbers, and the most troubling, of medical problems. These six are

- caffeine
- salt
- milk
- processed foods
- sugar
- fats

What makes this book distinct from all other nutrition and dietary health books is that, in simple, practical steps, it helps you to determine whether some of your medical problems are caused by foods you eat and, if so, shows you how to solve them.

Even if your current diet is one that you learned as a child was healthy and well-balanced, you may be eating or drinking some ordinary food that affects the way you feel adversely. Like other physicians of my generation (I went to medical school in the early 1960s), I was taught "the four-food-group theory" of good nutrition. "To recommend a healthy diet," I was told, "just tell your patients to take sensible portions each day from four food groups: (1) grains, (2) fruits/vegetables, (3) meat/fish, and (4) dairy products." This may have been good advice before fast-food chains and ready-to-eat packaged foods came onto the scene, but today it is most difficult to choose a healthy diet that way. Just compare the two diets in table 1, each of which contains "sensible" servings from the four food groups. The foods in Diet I tend to be high in fat, salt, and sugar, as well as low in fiber and common nutrients. The foods in Diet II contain small amounts of fat, salt, and sugar, plus ample fiber and nutrients.

Don't be scared off by the "health food" tone of Diet II. This type of diet can be varied sufficiently to appeal to every taste. The more common Diet I, of course, contains a multitude of fat- and sodium-laden convenience foods. Their effects are cumulative; when these foods are taken in excess they may cause you to feel unwell and eventually endanger your health. The American Cancer Society, American Diabetes Association, and American Heart Association all advise against excessive fat, salt, and sugar intake, and they all recommend more fiber- and nutrient-rich foods than the typical American eats today. This book will pinpoint the problems

Table 1

Two Approaches to the Four Food Groups

	Diet I	Diet II
GRAINS	Captain Crunch cereal, white bread	Seven-grain cereal, whole-wheat bread
FRUIT	Orange juice	One orange
VEGETABLES	Potato chips, canned corn	Baked potato, fresh corn on the cob
MEAT/FISH	Kentucky Fried Chicken, deep-fried shrimp	Lean meat or fish, kidney beans, tofu
DAIRY	Chocolate milk (whole), strawberry yogurt	Skim milk or soy milk, plain low-fat yogurt

you might be having owing to the fats, salt, sugar, caffeine, and dairy products in your diet. It will also describe the results of inadequate fiber consumption.

The dairy products and caffeine-containing beverages discussed may be your favorites, and what I have to say about them may elicit your resistance. People tend to enjoy these foods and drinks so much that they do not want to hear about the multiple medical problems they can cause. But the fact remains, as the examples of John and Robert demonstrate, that these two categories of substances can *cause* some medical problems and *exacerbate* others.

Can you change your eating habits without turning into a diet freak? Yes! Many of my patients do so each month, when it becomes obvious to them that the foods they have been eating cause them discomfort, distress, or disease. These people have found simple ways to avoid symptoms, ranging from vague anxiety to severe depression, from simple headaches to frequent migraines, from bothersome digestive problems to severe intestinal disease.

If only one dietary item is causing problems for you, you could make a healthful change relatively quickly and easily. On the other hand, the longer it takes to identify offending items, the more items there are, and the greater your attachment to them, the more time and determination you will need to adopt better eating habits. However, as you begin to feel better, you will be more eager to continue, and this will make change easier. Don't expect this book to induce instant success or to offer miracle "crutches." *Do* expect it to help you to avoid problem food and drinks and to reduce or eliminate troubling symptoms. Just possibly, it will help you achieve the wonderful feeling of vitality and good health.

I

Caffeine — Friend or Foe?

Do you have any of these problems?

Angina
Anxiety
Bed-wetting
Birth defects (pregnancy)
Breast tenderness
Cancer
Cystitis (urinary tract
   infection)
Depression
Diarrhea
Fast heart rate (tachycardia)
Fatigue
Fibrocystic breasts
Gastritis
Headaches
Heartburn
Heart disease
Heart palpitations
   (arrhythmias)

High blood pressure
High cholesterol level
Hyperactivity
Hypoglycemia
Insomnia
Itchy anus
Nightmares
Osteoporosis
Panic disorder
Premenstrual syndrome
Prostatitis
Rectal pain
Restlessness
Ringing in ears (tinnitus)
Throat lump (globus)
Tremors (shakiness)
Ulcers
Urethritis/trigonitis
Urinary frequency

If you answered yes and if you drink any caffeine, read
on to see how your health problems might be caused
or worsened by your caffeine consumption.

Chapter 1

The Harmful Effects of Caffeine

Might you or a member of your family be suffering needlessly because of excessive caffeine intake? Before you pooh-pooh that possibility on the grounds that no one in your family drinks more than a cup or two of coffee a day, consider that many popular foods, drinks, and medications contain as much caffeine per average serving as an average cup of coffee. Consider, too, that many people react symptomatically to relatively small quantities of caffeine. Some people are so sensitive to caffeine that even the barely measurable quantity used to flavor a frozen dairy dessert is enough to trigger symptoms.

Caffeine is a drug, and as with even the most useful drugs, it is not to be taken lightly. It is a powerful stimulant with substantial addictive potential. It belongs to a class of chemical compounds called methylxanthines, which are found naturally in more than sixty plant species. Its most familiar sources include coffee beans, tea leaves, cacao seeds (from which cocoa is made), and kola nuts (from which the cola flavoring used in many soft drinks is derived). Caffeine is often used in small quantities in flavoring agents for pastries, frozen dairy desserts, gelatin puddings, and soft candies.

Current Food and Drug Administration regulations do not require that caffeine in flavoring agents be labeled, since the quantities used per serving are often very small. Unfortunately for some people, a tiny amount is often too much. Such people may have great difficulty in isolating the products that are affecting them adversely.

Caffeine has many effects on the human body, not all of them bad. In fact, some effects of this substance are clearly beneficial:

- It promotes alertness,
  helping us wake up or stay awake.
- It enhances energy.
- It elevates low moods.
- It helps to relieve pain, particularly when used with
  aspirin or acetaminophen (e.g., Tylenol).

All these effects are due to caffeine's stimulation of the central nervous system (which includes the brain) or the cardiac muscle (heart).

As long as we don't consume too much caffeine and don't become sensitive or allergic to it, the benefits may seem to outweigh the drawbacks. However, caffeine has several harmful or highly unpleasant effects that may go unrecognized:

- It stimulates the central nervous system.
- It stimulates excessive gastric acid secretion.
- It relaxes smooth muscle (e.g., in the bladder).
- It stimulates heart muscle.
- It increases urine production.
- It raises the level of free fatty acids in the blood.
- It elevates blood glucose (sugar) levels.

Very few people need more acid in their stomach, more frequent or urgent urination, or more fats and sugar in their blood. Then why do so many people take in caffeine indiscriminately? Some of the reasons are that caffeine is relatively inexpensive, socially acceptable, easily obtainable, and heavily promoted. In one recent year, General Foods spent $57 million advertising and promoting its Maxwell House coffee.[1] Proctor & Gamble spent $27.5 million doing the same for its Folgers brand. The entire industry is bent on keeping its old friends drinking as much coffee as possible and on encouraging young people to start. Targeting the 18-to-34-year-old age group, advertisers feature popular idols—professional sports stars, actors, writers —savoring coffee in every imaginable situation. Small wonder that people overlook the addictive or otherwise harmful aspects of caffeine and search for another cause when adverse effects begin to manifest themselves.

If you have one of the problems described below, and if you and your physician have been unable to find an explanation for the symptoms, caffeine may be the culprit. Unless you suspect that immediate medical evaluation is indicated, a two-week trial of abstinence from caffeine is in order. This trial may eliminate all symptoms and return you to a sense of true well-being. At the very least, it may save you from a costly, roundabout way of learning the simple fact that excessive caffeine can cause you problems.

Anxiety, Hyperactivity, and Panic Disorders

Diane had lost her job eight months before her visit to me. She now had a new job that she enjoyed, but she continued to feel anxious, nervous, and restless. These symptoms had begun with the stress of losing her job, but she was concerned about the fact that they were continuing even now when "all seems well." Diane's anxiety symptoms disappeared entirely when she abstained from coffee drinking for two weeks. The symptoms returned if she drank even a single cup.

An intolerance to a food often begins during a stressful period in our life. Symptoms can occur not just after psychological stress of the sort Diane experienced, but also after physical stress such as a bad case of the flu or mononucleosis, a fatiguing school term, or even a stretch of excessive manual labor.

Feelings of apprehension, fear, tremors, or uncertainty without understandable cause may be the manifestation of a treatable illness called panic disorder. Often, such feelings are accompanied by rapid heartbeat, sweating, or nausea, all symptoms that can be traced directly to overuse of caffeine. Numerous studies have related caffeine use to an increased incidence of not only general anxiety symptoms but also panic disorders in adults and hyperactivity in children.[2] Imagine how helpful it would be to teachers and parents if some children were a bit less jumpy and restless. Hyperactive children may be showing the effects of the caffeine in the soft drinks and hot chocolate they like so much. Interestingly, in a minority of children caffeine has the opposite effect, actually calming them down.

Bed-Wetting

Psychological causes of nocturnal enuresis (bed-wetting) may not be uncommon, but they can be very difficult to isolate. Yet a child's bed-wetting problem may have a simple and easily remedied cause: too much caffeine. Take Danny, age 7, for example, who was wetting his bed about twice a week when his parents brought him to me. They had followed every one of their doctor's suggestions, including a consultation with a clinical psychologist, without success. Danny was in every other aspect an ideal child. He was loving and loved and popular with his siblings and his classmates. No one could find in his personality or habits any clinical cause of nocturnal enuresis.

When I questioned Danny's mother about his diet, she told me that Danny loved cocoa and often drank two cups or more with his meals. Eliminating cocoa, chocolate candy, and cola from Danny's diet stopped his bed-wetting completely. I have found no studies implicating caffeine as a cause of bed-wetting, but it has been an apparent cause a couple of times in my practice. A more common cause of bed-wetting is milk, discussed in part V.

Fatigue

Charles, a 44-year-old business manager, came to see me

because he was afraid he might have cancer, which both his father and his grandfather had had.

Charles told me he was tired all the time, really fatigued, without an ounce of his previous energy. He'd been asked to develop plans for a big new project in his company, and he just couldn't concentrate long enough to complete his plans. Besides feeling tired, he said he was nervous and jumpy, unable to sleep more than a couple of hours at a stretch. Very sensibly, he had turned to a friend who did professional counseling. The counselor recommended that he have a complete physical checkup, and Charles jumped to the conclusion that he might have cancer.

In investigating Charles's life-style, I learned that he had been divorced a year and half previously, without rancor and with a stressless financial settlement. The only unsettling aspect of the divorce, he said, was that he no longer followed a regular eating schedule. He would often skip breakfast and sometimes lunch, making do with only coffee, candy bars, and soft drinks on the job. His eating habits plus the two to four Excedrin tablets he took a day for frequent headaches had Charles taking in nearly 1,000 mg of caffeine on an average day—well above what most researchers call the danger level.[3]

I suggested that Charles hold off on an expensive cancer workup and try a fourteen-day abstinence from coffee, which would cost him nothing except perhaps some withdrawal pain. He agreed, and two weeks later on a follow-up visit he thanked me and said he was feeling great, sleeping soundly all night, and eager to put the finishing touches on his project's plans. He found it hard to believe that so many worrisome symptoms had been due primarily to caffeine, but he couldn't refute the results of his abstinence.

Cystitis, Urethritis, Trigonitis, and Prostatitis

Inflammation or infection of the urinary bladder (cystitis), bladder opening (trigonitis), urethra (urethritis), or prostate (prostatitis) is often accompanied by burning pain upon urination, low back ache, and/or low abdominal pains. These are frequently temporary conditions easily relieved by appropriate medications.

But for those who suffer recurrently, these are most aggravating problems. Before beginning a long medical workup, try a period of caffeine abstinence. It frequently works! Despite an absence of studies proving a connection between caffeine and these infections, many urologists and patients testify that eliminating caffeine often clears up a recurrent urinary tract or prostate infection.

Diarrhea

Loose, watery, and frequent stools can be a real nuisance, especially when one is 86 years old and has trouble getting around. One of my nursing-home patients, Mabel, had exactly this problem. She didn't complain, but her nurses did. Mabel began to soil her underclothes while trying to get to the bathroom. She reported no recent changes in her routine, so proctoscopy and lower bowel x-ray studies were done. All were quite normal.

Upon further questioning, Mabel admitted to drinking five or six cups of hot chocolate a day and to taking several Anacin tablets each day for arthritic pain. A friend was bringing her the hot chocolate mix and Anacin, both of which I had previously stopped because of suspected caffeine-caused insomnia. Finally, Mabel was convinced that caffeine *was* at fault; when she stopped taking it in, she went back to a normal bowel schedule.

This was especially interesting to me, because I had not been aware previously that caffeine consumption might be a cause of chronic diarrhea, although this connection has been reported.[4] Since then, knowledge of this fact has helped several of my patients avoid a lot of unnecessary bowel x-rays and stool exams. You can see why both my patients and I get excited when simple nutritional changes help them feel better and avoid unnecessary tests.

Ulcers, Gastritis, and Esophagitis

The type of burning stomach or chest pain that suggests a diagnosis of ulcers, gastritis, or esophagitis may be caused by excessive caffeine. Some patients who come to me with worries about ulcers or severe heartburn lose all symptoms after eliminating caffeine from their diets. Nick, for example, came to me after exhaustive efforts had failed to relieve his "ulcer pain" or to identify a clear reason for it. One doctor had prescribed an ulcer medication called Tagamet, he said, and that had worked for a while after a long string of antacids had failed.

When asked about coffee drinking, he cheerfully admitted to drinking ten to fifteen cups a day. "It's all that keeps me going on my long trucking hauls," he said. I told him that I thought it might be the cause of his pain, so he reluctantly agreed to try to live without it for a fourteen-day trial period. I told him to start during a long weekend at home, because suddenly giving up that amount of caffeine can cause painful withdrawal. He laughed at me, but the next afternoon called for help. "My head is killing me and I'm a bear with my kids," he said. I offered to give him a light sedative, but he said he didn't like to take that kind of medication and asked if I could suggest something else. "You might ask your wife to take the kids to visit Grandma, or find a quiet motel room for a day or so," I said.

Several weeks later Nick called to say he felt just great. His wife had had her mother come to stay with the kids for the weekend, and she had gone with him to a motel. "She needed a rest as much as I needed quiet. By Monday morning we both felt wonderful." He'd been on the road all week, he said, without any heartburn or stomach pain. When he felt really sleepy, he pulled into a rest stop. The absence of pain made the lack of coffee easy to deal with.

For years, doctors have debated whether caffeine increases inflammation of the esophagus, stomach, and duodenum. It seems to make sense that caffeine would cause problems there, because one of its normal actions is to stimulate acid secretion in the stomach. Most studies show that caffeine does not *cause* ulcers but may exacerbate preexisting conditions and increase symptoms.[5] I have found that a number of patients experience much relief from heartburn or stomach pains when they stop drinking both caffeinated and decaffeinated brews.

Fibrocystic Breast Disease

Despite inconclusive scientific evidence, my clinical experience convinces me that there must be a connection between caffeine and aggravated fibrocystic breast disease.[6] For example, Eleanor was a vibrant 26-year-old woman who came to see me for advice about mastectomy and reconstructive surgery "to get rid of my fibrocystic breast disease once and for all."

Eleanor's breasts were often painfully swollen for two weeks before her menstrual period, and she'd recently had a benign fibrous cyst removed surgically. An older sister with a history of lumps, biopsies, and constant fear of cancer had had a bilateral mastectomy and reconstruction with implants two years before. She elected this route to alleviate her constant worry. Eleanor's sister now felt a great deal better about her future. Eleanor wanted reassurance that a similar course could be right for her. Until recently, fibrocystic breasts were considered by many to be precancerous. We now know that the real problem is not that this condition will lead to cancer but that it will confuse the situation with recurrent lumps and produce anxiety in both patient and physician.

Exam and mammography indicated that Eleanor did indeed have fibrocystic breast disease, but major surgery seemed far too serious a step for immediate consideration. Her premenstrual breast pain might well have another source, I assured her; excessive caffeine might possibly be involved. She agreed to eliminate all caffeine-containing products for six months. "Is there anything else I can do?" she asked, and I told her that a moderate daily dose of vitamin E might be helpful. She agreed to take 200 IUs (international units) daily. Some evidence suggests that this vitamin can reduce cysts in the breasts, though the relationship has not been proven.

Six months later, Eleanor reported almost no premenstrual breast pain or swelling "for at least three months now." She had developed no new lumps, and the existing fibrocystic areas had not increased in size. She was extremely pleased at the prospect of a normal life despite her fibrocystic breast disease.

This doesn't mean that, if you have fibrocystic breast disease, you should simply give up caffeine and quit worrying. Any new lump, painful or not, deserves evaluation. My point is that in some women, caffeine seems to make fibrocystic lumps more painful or more frequent, and eliminating caffeine might help the problem considerably.

Osteoporosis

It is well known that adequate calcium is necessary for strong bones. Unfortunately, it is not well known by the public that calcium loss from urine doubles following caffeine consumption.[7] Studies by other researchers have agreed that caffeine causes us to lose calcium.

Those people with osteoporosis or at increased risk for its development should know that stopping caffeine consumption will help supply the body with more calcium, making bones stronger.

Headaches

Do you often have severe headaches for no apparent reason? Caffeine may be causing them. Mary, a 36-year-old guidance counselor balancing her career with wife-mother responsibilities, came to me for help after months of increasingly painful headaches. The headaches had become severe at about the time her teenage son was caught siphoning gasoline from a neighbor's car. Mary and her regular physician had assumed the headaches were related to stress involving the son's behavior, but several months later, when the youth's problems seemed totally resolved, Mary's headaches not only persisted but increased in severity. She was sent to a large medical center for neurologic evaluation, and extensive tests revealed nothing significant. She was given medication for tension headaches and told to avoid stressful activities as much as possible. The pills seemed to help sometimes, but at other times they did not help at all.

In my early conversations with Mary, I learned that she was an inveterate coffee drinker. She had grown up in a Scandinavian community, in a home where there was always fresh coffee on the stove, and had started drinking coffee at age 7. Now she usually consumed two to five cups a day.

In reviewing her headache-free periods in recent months, Mary recalled that she had felt fine for at least six days on an eight-day canoe trip in Northern Minnesota's Boundary Waters, although she'd had excruciating pain the first couple of days out. "Were you having your usual cups of coffee each day?" I asked. "No," she said, "no one remembered to bring coffee, so we had to do without it the whole eight days." When I suggested that her severe headaches on the first days of the trip may have been caused by caffeine withdrawal, she said, "Surely not." But then she remembered that she usually experienced her worst headaches on days when she drank very little coffee or was visiting someone who had nothing but decaffeinated coffee in the house.

Mary willingly tried a fourteen-day elimination of coffee. After three days of severe headaches, she was completely headache-free for the rest of the time. When she tried to have only a cup of coffee a day, because she really loved it, the headaches recurred. The elimination diet allowed her body to regain its sensitivity to coffee, and now responded with headaches to even the smallest amount. Now she avoids caffeine completely and carefully reads the label of every new medication or soft drink she considers buying.

Frequently, I have found that a major stress, such as that Mary experienced in dealing with her child's trouble, triggers intolerance to caffeine. Such intolerance may continue after the stress has passed. I suspect that Mary's variable coffee intake of five cups one day and two the next caused intermittent withdrawal headaches. Even if caffeine users do not report problems from stopping its use, they have been shown to have more headaches than abstainers.[8]

The elimination of caffeine intake for some and the reduction for others could result in considerable benefit for thousands of headache sufferers.

Cancer

If you are looking for controversy, this is where you can find it. Findings on whether caffeine causes cancer range from some studies showing a definite correlation to others showing a protective effect of caffeine against the same kind of cancer! Two cancers in particular that are surrounded with such conflicting findings are breast cancer and colon or rectal cancer? Other types of cancer for which some studies show an increased incidence with caffeine use are cancer of the pancreas, prostate, and urinary bladder.[10] Because of the controversy, it makes sense to me that all people should be careful of their caffeine intake. Those with a strong family history of cancer should probably be even more careful. My guess is that one or two cups of coffee each day will not be a problem for most people. Unfortunately, it is not uncommon for many of my patients to drink eight to twenty cups daily.

High Cholesterol (Hypercholesterolemia)

It's a little-known but well-proven fact that simply eliminating caffeine from the diet can lower the blood cholesterol level by up to 13 percent.[11] Moreover, every 1 percent drop in cholesterol is associated with a 2 percent drop in heart attack risk.[12] A very worried 48-year-old Peter came to me because two years on a low-fat diet prescribed by another doctor had lowered his cholesterol level only a little—from 290 to 260 mg/dl (less than 200 is considered ideal). He knew that high cholesterol was a risk factor for coronary disease, and his father had died of a heart attack at age 50.

Peter wasn't aware that the caffeine he was getting from seven to ten cups of coffee and a few diet colas a day was a factor in his cholesterol level. He agreed to stop consuming caffeine, add oat bran to his cereal each morning, include more whole-grain foods and fresh fruit in his diet, decrease his fat consumption even further, and take a brisk twenty-minute walk each day.

Peter followed this regimen conscientiously. In one year, his cholesterol level was down to 188! At the same time, his blood pressure readings went from an average of 149/90 to 126/84 (safe = 120–130/80–85) and his body fat fell from 25 percent to 20 percent (safe = 12–18 percent). "I haven't felt this good since

I was 20," Peter said, "and I really enjoy the food I eat and the exercise." In just one year, he had significantly reduced his risk of having a heart attack by at least 40 to 50 percent. Given Peter's results, the benefits of stopping caffeine certainly seem substantial.

Nightmares (Night Terrors or Night Panic)

Six-year-old Susan awoke screaming uncontrollably at least once a week, and each time it took her frightened parents ten to fifteen minutes to calm her. Mystified and worried, they came to see me. When Susan's caffeine intake was totaled, it was easy to understand her agitation. With every meal, she was having either hot chocolate (which contains 2 to 20 mg per five-ounce cup) or chocolate milk (5 to 7 mg per cup). She often had several chocolate chip cookies (2 to 10 mg each) between meals and one glass of Mountain Dew (55 mg per can). When all Susan's known sources of caffeine were stopped, she (and her parents) had no more sleepless nights.

I have been unable to find any studies relating nightmares to caffeine intake. However, it makes sense that there might be a relationship, since, as you will recall, one of caffeine's normal actions is to stimulate the central nervous system, whose main component is the brain. Once every few years, a mother will tell me that her child's nightmares stopped when caffeine-containing foods were stopped and that they recur if the child begins to eat these foods again. I believe a two-week trial period of abstinence from foods containing caffeine is well worth the trouble for any child or adult with nightmares.

Heart Disease (Heart Attack and Angina), High Blood Pressure (Hypertension), and Heart Arrhythmias (Tachycardia and Palpitations)

Premature atrial contractions (PACs) and premature ventricular contractions (PVCs) are common arrhythmias often referred to as palpitations by those experiencing them. While these may occasionally be symptoms of severe cardiac problems and should not be regarded casually, the cause may be quite simple.

Joan, 26, an up-and-coming administrative secretary, came to see me two months after her heart began "just palpitating for no reason at all." Nothing seemed to be amiss; her history, physical examination, and electrocardiogram (ECG) were all normal.

Had Joan recently changed her eating or drinking habits at all? Well, about two months ago her office had obtained a new drip coffeemaker, and because the coffee "tasted so much better" she'd gone from her usual two or three cups of instant coffee each day (60 mg of caffeine per cup) to about six cups of drip coffee (115 mg of caffeine per cup). Her daily intake had suddenly quadrupled, from about 150 mg to more than 600 mg. Joan quickly agreed to eliminate caffeine entirely for two weeks. By the third day she noted no abnormal heartbeats. On two or three occasions she went over a one-cup-a-day limit of coffee, and on each occasion she experienced PVCs. She no longer goes over the limit.

Again, it makes sense that caffeine will occasionally cause the extra heartbeats called heart arrhythmias, since one of its normal physiologic actions is to stimulate heart muscle. This stimulation to the heart can also cause people to have a racing heart, or tachycardia.

Can coffee cause heart attacks? Until recently the evidence was quite controversial. But a newly published study of medical students followed for nineteen to thirty-five years showed that men who drank more than four cups of coffee daily had almost *three times* the incidence of heart disease (heart attacks or angina) than those who did not drink coffee.[13] Even the men who drank one or two cups of coffee per day had twice the risk of heart disease. Studies such as this one have caused me to question my belief that one or two cups of coffee a day is all right for most people.

Since many people die suddenly from heart arrhythmias, we need to be concerned that coffee may not only increase heart attacks but may cause sudden and fatal disturbances of heart rhythm.

Another risk factor for heart disease is high blood pressure. Coffee drinking will usually increase blood pressure for one or two days. Then, said one study, a tolerance develops to the coffee, and by the third day the caffeine does not seem to affect blood pressure very much.[14] Another study disagreed, concluding that coffee consumption contributed significantly to increased blood pressure levels.[15]

These studies alone demonstrate the critical importance of what and how much we eat and drink. Heart disease is our number one health problem today. Major factors contributing to heart disease are high cholesterol, high blood pressure, heart arrhythmias, and hardening of the coronary arteries. Much evidence now supports the hypothesis that caffeine is a cause of or can aggravate these conditions.

Pregnancy and Birth Defects

If, after reading about all these potential problems, you are still drinking your coffee, the possibility of birth defects may be an area that will change your mind. Again, the evidence is controversial but frightening. In a group of almost 500 pregnant women, sixteen had a daily caffeine intake of 600 mg or greater (eight to ten cups of coffee). Of the sixteen, eight miscarried, five had stillbirths, and two had premature infants.[16] Only one of the sixteen heavy coffee drinkers had a normal pregnancy outcome.

What is really interesting is that problems occurred also in a large number of the pregnancies where the *fathers* consumed high levels of caffeine (600 mg or more daily). In the thirteen cases fitting this criterion, the mother took in less than 400 mg caffeine daily, but there were still four miscarriages, two stillbirths, and two premature births. Only five of these couples had uncomplicated deliveries.

The study found that in twenty-three households where both partners drank less than 450 mg of caffeine daily, there were *no* pregnancy complications. It seems that any couple considering pregnancy would be wise to look carefully at their caffeine intake.

High doses of caffeine have long been linked to birth defects in animals,[17] though research on humans has not shown a relationship between caffeine intake and birth defects. Nonetheless, prudent parents will probably not want to take chances, even if the evidence is not at all certain.

Hyperactivity, Insomnia, and Tremors

The relationship between caffeine intake and the common problems of hyperactivity, insomnia, and tremors is well known, so I will say little about these conditions here. But if you do not believe that these three problems are often caused by caffeine, check out the link for yourself. Go without any caffeine for a few days. Then drink about six cups of coffee in one hour. If you are like the majority of people, you will develop a slight hand tremor, become more nervous or "hyper," and have some trouble falling asleep.

Remember, the physiologic action of caffeine on the body is to stimulate the central nervous system. Since the brain and its sleep center are part of the nervous system, brain-related side effects can and often do occur.

Rectal Pain or Itching

A common problem my patients always hate to discuss with me is rectal pain or itching. They are afraid I will respond by doing a proctoscopic exam. They tend to discuss these discomforts only after they have endured them for months or years, to the point of "going crazy."

The rectal pain, called proctalgia fugax, is a severe, sharp pain that often awakens one in the middle of the night. It usually goes away in minutes and never lasts more than a half hour, but it tends to scare people a lot. Frequently, elimination of caffeine will stop the problem completely.[18]

Itching around the anus, called pruritus ani, is also a common problem. Almost once each week a patient will hesitantly discuss it. If specific causes such as fissures, hemorrhoids, and infection are ruled out by my exam, I will have the patient do two things:

- Avoid scented soaps, toilet paper, and bath oils.
- Avoid all caffeine for two weeks.

A great many people with pruritus ani find 100 percent relief by carrying out these two suggestions. In those who don't, I then evaluate intake of other foods, such as citrus fruits, apples, nuts, corn, and dairy products, any of which can cause anal itching. Overall, 70 percent of my patients with this complaint experience relief with simple dietary changes.

Other Problems

My patients have taught me that the symptoms and diseases listed below will sometimes improve or vanish with caffeine avoidance even though research has yet to confirm the relationship of these conditions to caffeine intake:

- depression
- hypoglycemia
- leg cramps at night
- lumps in the throat (globus)
- premenstrual syndrome (PMS)
- ringing in the ears (tinnitus)

You might have one of these problems and decide to give caffeine avoidance a trial. If it helps, it will have been a very inexpensive solution to what may have been a nagging problem.

Notes

1. S. Zuckerman, "A Desperate Industry Reaches Out to Halt a Long-Term Decline," *Nutrition Action* (April 1984).
2. D. S. Charney et al., "Increased Anxiogenic Effects of Caffeine in Panic Disorders," *Archives of General Psychiatry* 42 (March 1985): 233–43; R. N. Elkins et al., "Acute Effects of Caffeine in Normal Prepubertal Boys," *American Journal of Psychiatry* 138 (February 1981): 2; and K. Z. Bezchlibnyk et al., "Should Psychiatric Patients Drink Coffee?" *Canadian Medical Association Journal* 124 (15 February 1981): 357–58.
3. T. Ferguson and M. A. Graedon, "Caffeine," *Medical Self-Care* (Winter 1981).
4. A. Wald et al., "Effect of Caffeine on the Human Small Intestine," *Gastroenterology* 71 (1976): 738–42.
5. L. A. Turnberg, "Coffee and the Gastrointestinal Tract," *Gastroenterology* 75 (1978).
6. J. P. Minton et al., "Caffeine, Cyclic Nucleotides, and Breast Disease." *Surgery* (July 1979); and F. Lubin et al., "A Low-Control Study of Caffeine and Methylxanthines in Benign Breast Disease," *Journal of the American Medical Association* 253 (1985).
7. L. Massey, "Caffeine and Calcium Loss," *Modern Medicine* 13 (August 1986); R. P. Heaney and R. R. Recker, "Effects of Nitrogen, Phosphorus and Caffeine on Calcium Balance in

Women," *Journal of Laboratory Clinical Medicine* 99 (1982); and M. Noteloritz, "Osteoporosis Held Completely Preventable with Lifestyle Changes and Medical Therapy," *Family Practice News* 14 (1984).

8. M. J. Shirlow and C. D. Mothers, "A Study of Caffeine Consumption and Symptoms: Indigestion, Palpitations, Tremor, Headaches, and Insomnia," *International Journal of Epidemiology* (April–June 1985): 239–48.

9. F. Lubin et al., "Coffee and Methylxanthines and Breast Cancer: A Case-Control Study," *Journal of National Cancer Institute* 74 (March 1985): 569–648; and C. Garland, "Mild Association Reported Between Coffee Intake and Colorectal Cancer," *Family Practice News* 16 (1986): 26.

10. B. MacMahon et al., "Coffee and Cancer of the Pancreas," *New England Journal of Medicine* 304 (12 March 1981): 630–33; and P. Cole, "Coffee-Drinking and Cancer of the Lower Urinary Tract," *Lancet* (26 June 1981): 135–37.

11. A. H. Forde et al., "The Tromso Heart Study: Coffee Consumption and Serum Lipid Concentrations in Men," *British Medical Journal* 290 (23 March 1985): 893–95; and D. S. Thelle et al., "The Tromso Heart Study: Does Coffee Raise Serum Cholesterol?" *New England Journal of Medicine* 308 (16 June 1983): 1454–57.

12. M. Rees, "Review of Tromso Heart Study," *Modern Medicine* (October 1985): 96.

13. A. Z. LaCroix et al., "Coffee Consumption and the Incidence of Coronary Heart Disease," *New England Journal of Medicine* 315 (October 1986): 977–82.

14. D. Roberson et al., "Caffeine and Hypertension," *American Journal of Medicine* 77 (July 1984): 54–59.

15. T. Lang, et al., "Relation Between Coffee Drinking and Blood Pressure," *American Journal of Cardiology* 52 (December 1983): 1238–42.

16. P. S. Weathersbee et al., "Caffeine and Pregnancy," *Postgraduate Medicine* 62 (1977): 64–69.

17. H. Lee et al., "Toxic and Teratologic Effects of Caffeine on Explanted Early Chick Embryos," *Teratology* 25 (1982): 25; and E. Ritter et al., "Potentiative Interactions Between Caffeine and Various Teratogenic Agents," *Teratology* 25 (1982): 95–100.

18. C. Hines, "When Rectal Pain Has No Organic Cause," *Patient Care* (15 August 1986): 107.

Chapter 2

A Simple Test

If the preceding chapter gave you one or more reasons to suspect that caffeine might be causing you problems, there is a simple way to find out. Just stop taking any caffeine-containing foods for fourteen days. This is what is called an elimination diet. If you feel much better by the end of the fourteen-day trial, or if your symptoms have eased, then you probably had a caffeine-related problem.

If at the end of fourteen days you are not sure whether or not eliminating caffeine made any difference, you need to do what is called a rechallenge test. On day fifteen, you consume a large amount of caffeine—for example, six to ten cups of coffee. If your problem was caffeine related, the symptoms should reappear within the next twenty-four to forty-eight hours.

For example, if you have frequent headaches and are wondering if the headaches are caffeine related, stop all caffeine for fourteen days. Take note of whether you have headaches during the last few days of your trial elimination. If the headaches are caffeine-related, they should be better by this time. If you are not sure about a relationship by day fourteen, drink six to ten cups of coffee on day fifteen and be alert to headaches over the next one to two days. If your headaches return full force, there is a strong chance of a caffeine-headache connection. If no headache occurs, you had better start looking elsewhere for the cause of your headaches.

You won't be able to avoid tiny amounts of caffeine if you eat a lot of commercially prepared foods, but unless you're extremely sensitive to caffeine, those amounts will have no effect. Do stop consuming everything known to contain caffeine—coffee, chocolate, cocoa, tea, caffeine-labeled soft drinks, and certain medications. As you can see from tables 2, 3, and 4, caffeine is present in many substances. Interestingly, many drugs, such as weight-control aids and cold remedies, are becoming caffeine-free as the side effects of caffeine become more publicized.

Table 2

Caffeine Content of
Several Common Beverages and Foods

Item	Milligrams caffeine	
	Average	Range
Coffee (5-oz. cup)		
Brewed, drip	115	60–180
Brewed, percolator	80	40–170
Instant	65	30–120
Decaffeinated, brewed	3	2–5
Decaffeinated, instant	2	1–5
Tea (5-oz. cup)		
Brewed, major U.S. brands	40	20–90
Brewed, imported brands	60	25–110
Instant	30	25–50
Iced (12-oz. glass)	70	67–76
Cocoa beverage (5-oz. cup)	4	2–20
Chocolate milk beverage (8 oz.)	5	2–7
Milk chocolate (1 oz.)	6	1–15
Dark chocolate, semi-sweet (1 oz.)	20	5–35
Baker's chocolate (1 oz.)	26	26
Chocolate flavored syrup (1 oz.)	4	4

Source: U.S. Food and Drug Administration, Food Additive Chemistry Evaluation Branch, as reproduced in U.S. Food and Drug Administration, "The Latest Caffeine Scorecard," FDA Consumer (March 1984): 14. Based on evaluations of existing literature on caffeine levels.

Table 3

Caffeine Content of
Various Soft Drinks (12-oz. Servings)

Brand	Milligrams caffeine
Sugar-Free Mr. PIBB	58.8
Mountain Dew	54.0
Mello Yello	52.8
TAB	46.8
Coca-Cola	45.6
Diet Coke	45.6
Shasta Cola	44.4
Shasta Cherry Cola	44.4
Shasta Diet Cola	44.4
Mr. PIBB	40.8
Dr. Pepper	39.6
Sugar-Free Dr. Pepper	39.6
Big Red	38.4
Sugar-Free Big Red	38.4
Pepsi-Cola	38.4
Aspen	36.0
Diet Pepsi	36.0
Pepsi Light	36.0
RC Cola	36.0
Diet Riet	36.0
Kick	31.2
Canada Dry Jamaica Cola	30.0
Canada Dry Diet Cola	1.2

Source: Institute of Food Technologist (IFT) as reproduced in U.S. Food and Drug Administration, "The Latest Caffeine Scorecard," FDA Consumer (March 1984): 15. Based on data from National Soft Drink Association, Washington D.C., April 1983.

Table 4

Caffeine Content of
a Few Commonly Used Drugs

Caffeine is an ingredient in more than 1,000 nonprescription drug products as well as numerous prescription drugs. Most often it is used in weight control remedies, alertness or stay awake tablets, headache and pain relief remedies, cold products, and diuretics. When caffeine is an ingredient, it is listed on the product label. Some examples of caffeine-containing drugs are:

PRESCRIPTION DRUGS	*Milligrams caffeine*
Cafergot (for migraine headache)	100
Fiorinal (for tension headache)	40
Soma Compound (for pain relief, muscle relaxant)	32
Darvon Compound (for pain relief)	32

NONPRESCRIPTION DRUGS	
Alertness tablets	
NoDoz	100
Vivarin	200
Analgesic/pain relief drugs	
Anacin, Maximum Strength Anacin	32
Excedrin	65
Midol	32
Vanquish	33
Diuretics	
Aqua Ban	100
Maximum Strength Aqua-Ban Plus	200

Source: FDA's National Center for Drugs and Biologics, as reproduced in U.S. Food and Drug Administration, "The Latest Caffeine Scorecard," FDA Consumer (March 1984): 16.

Avoiding caffeine can sometimes require a careful reading of all labels. Taking just half a cup of coffee or a chocolate candy bar during the withdrawal period may block your body's ability to reverse symptoms or problems caused by caffeine. Be sure to be strict with yourself for the entire two weeks.

Eliminating caffeine may be a *simple* solution but it is not always an *easy* one. It can be very difficult to withdraw from a substance to which your body has become accustomed and possibly addicted. A few basic tips will ease the elimination process for you. In just one or two days of total abstinence, your body will be caffeine-free, but that doesn't mean you'll be rid of caffeine's effects immediately. Withdrawal symptoms often persist for three days and may last as long as seven. You may not begin to feel truly well until your fourteen-day trial is nearly over.

Since caffeine is a strong drug, the withdrawal symptoms can be frightening. They're not as fearsome as those associated with alcoholism or so-called hard-drug addiction, and they don't persist as long, but they're just as real. My patients and I find that taking a good multiple vitamin-mineral supplement with each meal and an extra gram of vitamin C every day for about two weeks reduces the severity of caffeine-withdrawal symptoms. I also feel it's important to keep sugar consumption low and to get as much rest as possible, especially during the first few days of abstinence.

Some bizarre feelings can surface during the elimination. For example, Bill, a businessman in his forties, called me on the third day of his abstinence because he was afraid he was having a mental breakdown. He just couldn't stop crying; tears kept welling up and running down his cheeks. He told me he hadn't cried openly for more than thirty years, and he found it extremely embarrassing. It was a Friday; Bill had stopped a ten-cup-a-day coffee habit cold turkey three days before to be reasonably sure of being through withdrawal by an important business golf date on Sunday. I advised him to go home and go to bed for forty-eight hours, just as he would with a severe cold. By Sunday, he was beginning to feel fine, and he had no further problems of withdrawal. By the end of his fourteen-day trial, he was in lasting good spirits.

Depression severe enough to cause constant crying is extremely unusual in caffeine withdrawal, but you may feel one or more of the following to some extent (these symptoms are given in alphabetical order, because there's no rhyme or reason to their incidence):

- constipation
- depression
- disorientation
- fatigue
- headache
- irritability
- nausea
- sluggishness

Some people prefer to taper caffeine use for two to twelve weeks before undertaking the two-week abstinence test. This may well reduce the severity of withdrawal symptoms, perhaps even eliminating them entirely. To taper off, you may gradually lessen the number of cups of coffee and/or tea you drink daily and drink only caffeine-free soda. You might try having only decaffeinated coffee after breakfast or substituting caffeine-free drinks such as herb tea at lunch or snack times.

Decaffeinated Beverages

During total abstinence, you may still want a hot drink at breakfast time. Here are some good caffeine-free substitutes:

- bouillon or any meat broth
- grain-based beverages (Caffix, Postum, and Pero are common brands)

- herb tea (but read the label to be sure there's no caffeine)
- lemon-flavored hot water (use juice or peel)
- miso broth
- soy milk

Not all of these substitutes will appeal to you, but nearly everyone finds at least one of them palatable, and many people become devoted to their choices.

A fourteen-day elimination trial and challenge will be helpful only in determining whether certain of your symptoms or problems are caffeine related. Those problems most often helped by caffeine elimination are headaches, anxiety, fatigue, heart palpitations, gastritis, heartburn, hyperactivity, insomnia, anal itching, tremors, urinary frequency, and ringing in the ears.

Diseases such as heart disease, angina, and osteoporosis are long-term diseases. Evaluating whether caffeine elimination has helped reduce or cure them is difficult. For the long-term problems, we must go on our belief in studies and on faith. The studies showing significantly increased heart problems and osteoporosis in caffeine users make it quite easy to believe that avoidance or minimal use of caffeine will be helpful. And common sense helps us have faith that a substance we know can cause so many problems might cause some diseases (e.g., heart problems or osteoporosis) for which no empirical proof of the link exists.

So, go ahead! Give it a try! If you find even one symptom in chapter 1 that pertains to you, it is time to gear up for the fourteen-day caffeine-elimination trial. You might just be surprised at how well you feel afterward.

What You Can Expect

Are decaffeinated coffees and teas acceptable substitutes for people who are able to tolerate them in reasonable quantities?

Perhaps. The $64,000 question is, What is a reasonable quantity? As with caffeine, we don't really know whether even small amounts of daily decaffeinated brews over a long period are harmful.

Most coffee processors use a decaffeination process similar to the original one devised by Dr. Ludwig Roselius in Germany in 1908.[1] The coffee beans are steamed to draw the caffeine to the surface; a chemical solvent is then cycled through the beans for twelve to eighteen hours, removing approximately 97 percent of the caffeine. The beans are then steamed again to rinse the chemical.

In 1979, the Swiss developed a water-only decaffeination process. It used chemical solvents in making the product called Coffex (not to be confused with the grain-based beverage Caffix).[2] Coffex is made only in Switzerland by a process involving hot water and filtration with activated charcoal. Coffex is more expensive than other decaffeinated coffees, is sometimes difficult to find, and is slightly less flavorful than other brands. Now Nestlé and General Foods also have water-processed decaffeinated brews.

The chemical agents used over the years to decaffeinate the coffee bean strike fear into many food lovers. Agents used in the past include the following:

- benzene
- chloroform
- acetone
- trichlorethylene (TCE)
- ethyl alcohol
- ethyl ether
- formaldehyde

These seven have been gradually abandoned as better agents are developed or as reports filter in about negative side effects. One study, for example, showed that TCE caused cancer in mice.[3]

The two chemical agents now used most commonly for

decaffeinating coffee beans are methylene chloride and ethyl acetate. Ethyl acetate is used for High Point brand. Sanka brand was using methylene chloride until 1986, when they began to

Table 5

Decaffeinating Agents Used
in Specific Decaf Brands

BRANDS USING METHYLENE CHLORIDE
General Foods
  Brim
  Maxwell House
  Yuban
Chock-Full-o'-Nuts
Melitta
Tethy Foods
  Browned Gold
  Bustello
  El Pico
  Martinson
  Medalia D'Oro
  Savarin

BRANDS USING ETHYL ACETATE
Proctor & Gamble
  Folgers
  High Point

BRANDS USING WATER AND NATURAL OILS
Nestlé
  Nescafé
  Taster's Choice
General Foods
  Sanka

Source: "Methylene Chloride in Decaf Coffee Causes Concern but Alternatives Do Exist," Environmental Nutrition *(September 1986): 9.*

decaffeinate by water and carbon dioxide processing only.[4] This switch to water was probably an excellent idea, because methylene chloride has recently come under close scrutiny. This substance is an industrial solvent that is the active ingredient in a widely used paint remover. It is structurally related to chemicals known to cause cancer of the liver and pancreas in mice and rats. You can understand why people were beginning to have some concerns. Table 5 lists some brands and the agents used to decaffeinate them.

In fairness, nearly all authorities agree that a cup or two a day of decaffeinated brew will probably not cause harm to anyone. The habitual use of greater quantities is highly questionable, however, especially for pregnant women and nursing mothers. Anyone who drinks more than two to three cups a day is probably running unnecessary risks. In my experience, long-term use of any chemical or drug increases the chances of detrimental side effects.

The safest answer regarding intake of caffeinated or decaffeinated beverages is to limit yourself to one or two cups daily if you have any at all. If you drink more than this, a "caffeine fast" two days a week is a good way to avoid or check on possible addictive and withdrawal effects. Remember, pregnant women and nursing mothers are well advised to stay away from both caffeinated and decaffeinated products. The possible risks simply aren't worth taking. The rest of us can probably enjoy an occasional lift from caffeinated or decaffeinated beverages.

Notes

1. R. Kirschman, "The Search for Safe Decaf," *Medical Self-Care* (Winter 1983): 46–47
2. K. Johnson, "The Dangers of Decaf," *East West Journal* (August 1986): 14.
3. All data in the paragraph is from Kirschman, "The Search for Safe Decaf."
4. E. M. Grossman, "General Foods Letter to Physicians," personal correspondence, 2 February 1987.

II

Salt—
Is It Worth the Taste?

Do you have any of these symptoms or problems?

Bloating
Breast tenderness
Constipation
Cravings for liquids
Edema
Fatigue
Frequent urination
Headaches
Hemorrhoids

High blood pressure
Hypertension
Premenstrual syndrome
 (PMS)
Puffy feet and ankles
 (edema)
Ringing in ears (tinnitus)
Weakness

If you do have one of these problems, it is possible that the salt you are eating is the cause. Read on to learn more about salt.

Chapter 3

The Effects of Too Much Salt

Craig Claiborne, a well-known gourmet cook, found out that he had high blood pressure. In his book *Craig Claiborne's Gourmet Diet*, he describes how he decided to take the advice of his physician and go on a low-salt diet.[1]

Besides lowering his blood pressure from 186/112 to 140/80 (the safe range, you'll remember, is 120–130/80–85), Claiborne's lowering of his salt intake also had other wonderful effects. His hands, which had been red and puffy, returned to normal, he lost his chronic thirst, he lost twenty pounds, he acquired a sharper taste for foods, and he could walk without fatigue and shortness of breath. As Claiborne learned very quickly, salt can do *plenty* to your body. Actually, it is the sodium in salt that both helps the body (in small amounts) and hurts it (in the excess amounts we often eat).

Salt's scientific name is sodium chloride. The sodium component makes up 40 percent of salt; thus, 1,000 mg of salt contains 400 mg of sodium. People are often confused by discussions of amounts of salt and sodium. In this book, I refer to *sodium* content rather than salt content, since food packages are now labeled that way. Remember to check for the word *sodium* when searching for a food's salt content.

I learned in medical school that we humans need about 220 mg of sodium daily to function well. To be on the safe side, authorities have set guidelines well above that amount. So, the recommended daily allowance (RDA) is 1,000 to 3,000 mg. But guess what our average daily intake of sodium is in the United States. It is 4,000 to 8,000 mg—twenty to forty times more than what we really need and about four times more than the already-inflated RDA.

Is it any wonder that 20 to 40 million people in the United States have elevated blood pressure? If you take a finely tuned closed-system water pump and add an extra one or two quarts of water to it, that pump will have to work a lot harder to continue pumping the water. The blood in our circulatory system is composed primarily of water and works in much the same way. When we ingest extra salt, it brings more water out of our intestines and into our circulatory systems, thus forming more blood. Many things then happen to our bodies that are neither helpful nor healthy.

High Blood Pressure

Extra blood in the circulatory system makes the heart pump harder. This could be one factor in the development of hypertension. The exact manner in which sodium causes elevated blood pressure in some people is still not firmly established.[2] Besides making the heart pump harder by forcing it to push more blood through the system, excess sodium can increase the stiffness and rigidity of the arteries themselves.[3]

Not all people with high salt intake will develop elevated blood pressure. Evidence now suggests that only about 20 to 30 percent of the population is sensitive to sodium.[4] The remaining 70 to 80 percent of people do not seem to develop hypertension even with a large sodium intake. As you will see, that does not guarantee that excess sodium will not have other adverse effects on the body.

Constipation and Hemorrhoids

The stools often become more firm and bowel movements less frequent when salt intake is excessive. With excess salt intake, fluid in the intestine (which keeps stools soft) is drawn into the salty blood in the circulatory system. Constipation may then occur, which will cause straining at defecation and eventually hemorrhoids. Despite what you have learned about one stool a day being normal, people who begin to follow a low-sodium, high-fiber diet usually have two to four soft stools daily.

Frequent Urination

Excess sodium will cause an imbalance in such body minerals as potassium and chloride. The kidneys will then attempt to rebalance the minerals by removing the excess sodium (and manufacturing more and more urine). Consequently, people on high-sodium diets may urinate frequently; some of my patients report urinating up to fourteen times daily.

Liquid Cravings

Because we urinate frequently while trying to rebalance the body's minerals, we develop an excessive thirst. Unfortunately, we then often choose fluids that are not healthful, such as soft drinks, coffee, and alcohol. (The bartender serves free salted peanuts and popcorn with our drinks for a reason.) The liquid consumption of people who begin to eat primarily low-salt, high-fiber natural foods drops to an amazing degree. I have had patients call me to ask what was wrong with them because they were drinking only one or two glasses of fluid daily after changing to a whole-foods diet. I believe that with a diet very low in sodium and rich in high-fiber foods (fruits, grains, and vegetables), people probably do not need to drink more than one or two cups of liquids daily. There have been no studies proving this, but it may be that no one needs the six or eight glasses of fluids now recommended by doctors. No one really knows how much fluid we need to drink to be healthy. Try a true low-salt, high-fiber diet for a few weeks and observe what happens to your fluid intake.

Edema, Swelling, and Bloating

It makes sense that if one or two quarts of extra fluid are circulating in the system, some of it may leak out. This is exactly what happens.

I have many patients like Maude. When she was in for a yearly checkup and Pap smear, she said that her only problem was puffiness, especially in her feet and ankles. When I asked her about salt intake, she said she did not use it at all. When we looked over her three-day dietary analysis, it became clear that Maude was consuming 3,200 mg of sodium daily. You will recall that I said our bodies need only 220 mg of sodium daily. Maude was eating fourteen times the amount of sodium she really needed, and almost all of it was coming from hidden sources in packaged and processed foods.

If you feel bloated, puffy, and swollen, you may be able to lose ten pounds of water weight simply by trying a truly low-sodium diet.

Headaches

The universal malady called headaches is one of the more rewarding problems patients present to me, because it is one I can often help them solve through simple dietary methods. As you already know from chapter 1, many headaches are relieved by eliminating caffeine.

Another major cause of headaches is salt. In 1980, I read a book about salt-caused migraine headaches.[5] What fascinated me most was that the book was written by a surgeon. Surgeons, of course, do not deal much with headache problems, so I was interested to find out why this surgeon decided to write a book about headaches.

It turned out that Dr. Brainard, the author, had a long history of severe migraine headaches himself. He finally discovered that they tended to occur mainly if he consumed highly salted foods. He began to ask those of his surgery patients who also had migraines to try a low-salt diet. Many returned very enthusiastic, saying that the low-sodium diet had nearly stopped their migraine attacks. Dr. Brainard wanted to pass on this information to migraine sufferers, so he wrote the book.

Besides triggering migraine headaches, the overconsumption of dietary salt can cause the more common tension headaches. These headaches are often characterized by a generalized soreness or pain over the entire head, especially the temple area. I assume that, just as excess fluid leaks into body tissues causing edema and puffiness, so fluid leaks out around the brain, causing pressure and pain in the head. Thus, even if you don't have migraines but suffer from the more vague head pains we call tension headaches, a two-week low-salt trial diet would be worth a try.

Premenstrual Syndrome (PMS) & Breast Tenderness

Hormonal changes prior to menstruation bring more fluid into a woman's system. This is often the proverbial straw that breaks the woman's back. A woman may already have excess fluid in her body all month because of high salt consumption, but she may have learned to live with it. The hormone-induced extra fluid two to fourteen days before menses, however, is just too much. It puts pressure on her brain (causing irritability and mood swings), extra fluid in her breasts (causing breast pain) and ankles (causing edema), and makes her feel very fatigued. Do these symptoms sound familiar? If so, they could be in large part due to your salt intake!

PMS is a group of symptoms that occur in a cyclical manner in the days before menstruation. The reason why it affects some women and not others is unknown. My work since 1981 with hundreds of women having PMS convinces me that its causes are multifactorial, not nutritional alone. It is important to evaluate the emotional, social, mental, spiritual, and physical aspects of the woman's life as well as her genetic makeup. All these need to be explored and worked on. In the physical realm, as you have already seen, caffeine and salt can be two major factors causing PMS.

Fatigue, Weakness, and Tinnitus

Many of my patients who begin a low-salt diet discover amazing things. One of their best discoveries is a feeling of more energy and strength. Typically, they return for their checkups marveling at how much better they feel. A common comment is "Doc, I didn't even known I was so tired and weak."

Another rewarding finding is that salt reduction sometimes relieves the condition known as tinnitus, a constant ringing in the ears. Patients with this complaint are usually assured that they have no brain tumors or ear problems and are sent away with the depressing news that nothing can be done. "Live with it," is the usual advice. The patients I see with tinnitus assume that their problem is caused by high blood pressure, but it rarely is. Amazingly, when many of these people go on a low-salt diet, the tinnitus disappears. Neither I nor the medical literature have an explanation for this phenomenon.

You should now be aware that even if you have normal blood pressure, excess dietary salt can cause numerous problems or symptoms. You are also learning that even if you never use salt in cooking or at the table, you are probably consuming an excess amount from packaged and processed foods.

Let's explore where that salt is hiding.

Notes

1. C. Claiborne, *Craig Claiborne's Gourmet Diet* (New York: Ballantine, 1980).
2. "Salt and High Blood Pressure," *Consumer Reports* (March 1979): 147.
3. A. P. Avolio et al., "Improved Arterial Distensibility in Normotensive Subjects on a Low-Salt Diet," *Arteriosclerosis* (6 March 1986): 166.
4. J. Graedon, "Self-Medication," *Medical Self-Care* 17 (March 1986).
5. J. B. Brainard, *Control of Migraine* (New York: Norton, 1979).

Chapter 4

The Hidden-Salt Phenomenon

Chris's dad and uncle had high blood pressure, so Chris was aware of the importance of salt restriction and thought he was being quite careful about the amount of salt he ate. He never added salt at the table and his wife used it only rarely in cooking.

When eating breakfast out with a friend one morning, Chris watched smugly as his friend ordered three slices of bacon, two eggs, a piece of toast, and orange juice. Chris virtuously had a bowl of All-Bran cereal with milk, two English muffins with margarine, and tomato juice. Who do you think consumed more sodium, Chris or his friend? I'll keep you in suspense for a few minutes while I offer more details about salt.

Give a salty food to a small baby and you will most likely see the baby grimace or spit. Likewise, people from cultures with traditionally low-salt diets generally find salty foods distasteful. However, if salt is gradually introduced into their diet, they will often develop a craving for it. Our bodies can be taught some bad habits; unfortunately, that is what addiction is all about.

Salt is the second most popular food additive, ranking only behind sugar. Salt was originally added to foods primarily as a preservative. As our taste for it blossomed, it was added in larger and larger amounts as a flavor-enhancer. Food-processing companies now argue that the amount of salt they add to their products is based strictly on consumer demand. In fact, until the 1980s salt was heavily added to baby foods so that we parents would like it when we tried a little bit as we fed the baby!

Salt in very large amounts is hidden in most processed foods, even in those that don't taste salty. In fact, 75 percent of the salt in our diets comes from the salt added by the manufacturers to processed foods.[1] For example, ten (1 oz.) salty-tasting potato chips contain 130 mg of sodium, while just three 4-inch Aunt Jemima pancakes (which don't taste salty at all) contain 550 mg.

The well-intentioned Chris, described earlier, was not aware of this "hidden-salt phenomenon." The breakfast his friend ordered contained only 500 mg of sodium, while Chris's contained 1,300 mg. You may say that just doesn't seem right, especially since the friend even had salty bacon. Before analyzing these two breakfasts in terms of sodium content, I must make it clear that the friend's breakfast contained excess fat and cholesterol and in no way would I recommend such a meal. The example is intended to show how easily salt can be hidden, even in the food we often consider healthful. Take a look at table 6 for a sodium breakdown of the two meals.

Take a look at *your* sodium intake, using table 7 as a guide. The foods in the three groups shown in the table are those that many believe should be the core foods of our diet. Indeed, the majority of our distant ancestors ate mostly grains, vegetables, and fruit, a diet I myself believe suits our biological needs. As you can see, unless these foods are canned or packaged, they contain almost no salt. Even if we added certain meats to the

Table 6

The Sodium Content of Two Breakfasts

The friend's breakfast	Mg	Chris's breakfast	Mg
Bacon (3 strips)	240	All-Bran cereal	
Eggs (2)	122	(⅓ cup)	260
Toast (1 slice)	148	Milk (½ cup)	60
Orange juice (8 oz.)	2	Muffins (2)	402
		Margarine (2 pats)	92
		Tomato juice (8 oz.)	486
Total	512	Total	1,300

list (see table 8), the diet composed from those groups would be extremely low in sodium. But beware of the meats on table 9!

Table 7

The Sodium Content of Some Common Foods

Foods	Amount	Sodium (mg)
VEGETABLES		
Fresh (most varieties)	½ cup	0–40
Frozen	½ cup	0–40
Canned	½ cup	230–460
V-8 or tomato juice	½ cup	250–350
Celery, beets	½ cup	75
FRUITS		
Fresh or canned	½ cup	0
Fruit juice		
(most varieties)	½ cup	0
GRAINS		
Rice, macaroni, noodles	½ cup	0
Hot cereals (examples)		
Instant	1 oz.	0
Instant flavored	1 oz.	200
Quick	1 oz.	80
Cold cereals (examples)		
Shredded Wheat	½ cup	0
All-Bran	⅓ cup	260
Corn flakes, Cheerios	1 oz.	290
Grape Nuts	¼ cup	190

Source: The figures are approximations based on data in U.S. Department of Agriculture, Sodium Content of Foods, Handbook 456 (Washington, D.C.: U.S. Government Printing Office, 1985). For a copy write to the Office of Governmental and Public Affairs, Room 507A, U.S. Department of Agriculture, Washington, D.C. 20250.

Table 8
Low-Sodium Meats

Meats	Amount	Sodium (mg)
Beef, lamb, pork	1 oz.	20–30
Chicken, turkey, veal	1 oz.	20–30
Hamburger	3 oz.	46
Bacon, crisp	1 strip	80

Table 9
High-Sodium Meats

Meats	Amount	Sodium (mg)
Ham	1 oz.	288
Pork sausage	1 oz.	276
Hot dog	1	460
Bacon, Canadian	1 oz.	690

Unfortunately, the low-salt grains, vegetables, and fruits do not make up the bulk of what we Americans typically eat. Lunch foods, for example, especially for our children, often come from the list in table 10. And for the evening meal people often heat up a frozen or canned dinner from the bottom half of the table.

Often in a busy family there is no time to do any home cooking. What happens when we eat a meal out at a fast-food restaurant? We might be able to get a food from each of the four food groups, but *you* decide if these meals seem healthy. Don't even think about the fats and sugars yet. Just look at the sodium. Let's try a McDonald's meal for starters. Table 11 tells us that McDonald's has just given us 1,755 mg of sodium! Remember, you need 220 mg daily to do just fine. As table 12 shows, other fast-food selections rival the selections from

Table 10

Common High-Sodium Lunch and Dinner Foods

Foods	Amount	Sodium (mg)
Lunch		
Tuna salad sandwich	1	400–600
Tossed salad, dressing, croutons	1	400–600
Luncheon meat sandwich	1	570–670
Macaroni and cheese	1 cup	746
Campbell's canned soup	1 cup	800–930
Spaghetti with meat	1 cup	730–1,100
Chef Boyardee Beefaroni	1 cup	1,200
Dinner		
Pot pie	8 oz.	900–1,670
TV dinner (with meat)	12 oz.	850–1,775
Pizza, frozen or mix (14")	½	1,200–1,800
Morton king-size turkey dinner	1	2,600
Sloppy joe mix (dry, no meat)	1½ oz.	3,565

Table 11

The Sodium Content of a Typical Meal at McDonald's

Food	Amount	Sodium (mg)
Big Mac	1	955
French fries	20	100
Chocolate shake	1	300
Apple pie	1	400

Source: M. Franz, Fast Food Facts: Nutrition and Exchange Values for Fast Food Restaurants (Minneapolis: International Diabetes Center, 1985).

Table 12

Sodium Totals for Common Fast-Food Meals

Food	Amount	Sodium (mg)
Whopper (Burger King)	1	1,000
Ham and cheese (Arby's)	1	1,745
Chicken breast sandwich (Arby's)	1	1,323
Kentucky Fried Chicken (side breast, leg, keel)	3 pieces	1,396

Table 13

Sodium-Containing Compounds

COMPOUND	USE
Baking soda (sodium bicarbonate or bicarbonate of soda)	For leavening in the preparation of breads and cakes; sometimes added to vegetable cookery; as an alkalizer for indigestion
Baking powder	In the preparation of breads and cakes
Brine (salt and water solution)	In the processing of foods and in canning, freezing, and pickling
Disodium phosphate	In some quick-cooking cereals and processed cheeses
Monosodium glutamate (MSG)	As a seasoning in home and restaurant cooking and in many packaged, canned, and processed frozen foods

COMPOUND	USE
Sodium acetate	For pH control
Sodium alginate	For smooth texture in chocolate milks and ice creams
Sodium aluminum sulfate	For leavening
Sodium benzoate	As a preservative in condiments
Sodium calcium alginate	For smooth texture or thickening
Sodium citrate	For pH control
Sodium diacetate	As a preservative
Sodium erythorbate	As a preservative
Sodium hydroxide	In the processing of some fruits and vegetables, hominy, and ripe olives
Sodium nitrate	As a preservative
Sodium propionate	As a preservative
Sodium sorbate	As a preservative
Sodium stearyl fumarate	As a maturing and bleaching agent or dough conditioner
Sodium sulfite	As a bleach for some fresh fruits and as a preservative in some dried fruits

Source: L. Hachfield, "Sodium Containing Compounds," unpublished report personal communications.

McDonald's. And you haven't even added the sodium in your fries, potato salad, or shake.

A multitude of salt-containing substances are used in prepared foods. These are other hidden sources of sodium that can fool even the careful label reader. Table 13 lists common sodium-containing compounds and their uses in the processed-food industry.

As our friend Chris found out when he tried to watch his salt intake, salt is everywhere and is very well hidden. How can you kick the salt habit? Read on!

Notes

1. W. P. T. James et al., "The Dominance of Salt in Manufactured Food in the Sodium Intake of Affluent Societies," *Lancet* 1 (February 1987): 426.

Chapter 5

Eating Well While Sparing the Salt

A patient named Donna explained to me that ever since her thirtieth birthday three years before, she could hardly stand herself the week before her menstrual period. Her breasts would be swollen and sore, she would feel bloated and irritable, and she would have lots of headaches. After a thorough medical evaluation, I had Donna chart her symptoms for three months. This confirmed her belief that the problems primarily occurred in the one week before menstruation, a problem called premenstrual syndrome (PMS). I suggested that she see our nutrition counselor. During two or three sessions with the dietician, Donna learned how to change her diet easily to include less salt—an important treatment for PMS. After three months on her new dietary program, she happily reported that all of her premenstrual symptoms were at least 50 percent improved.

Donna's success with salt limitation inspired her to make further dietary changes—namely, to cut down on the excessive fats and sugars she was eating. She said she would not have believed before she changed her eating habits that decreasing the salt in her diet could have made so much difference.

Like Donna (and Chris, and Craig Claiborne, mentioned previously), you can decrease your salt intake quite easily by 50 percent to 70 percent. Try it for two or three months and observe the changes. Your average blood pressure reading may decrease, even if it is within the normal range before you begin. Premenstrual symptoms will probably decrease in intensity. You will have more energy and less bloating and puffiness. You may have fewer headaches. Even your bowels may work better!

Remember, average daily sodium intake in the United States is 6,000 mg/day. The salt you add to foods in cooking and at the table accounts for only about one-sixth of that, or 1,000 mg. So, if you stop adding salt in cooking or at the table, you are doing something, but not yet enough to make a significant difference.

One-tenth of our daily salt intake (600 mg) comes from the sodium naturally contained in foods. For instance, one 8-ounce glass of milk contains 120 mg of sodium. You can see that if a child drinks two quarts of milk per day (as some do!), he or she is taking in 960 mg of sodium without even touching a "salty" food.

Let's review where our 6,000 mg of sodium comes from each day:

- Added in cooking or at the table: 1,000 mg
- Contained naturally within foods: 600 mg

Where do the other 4,400 mg of sodium come from? Having read chapter 4, you realize now that much of the remaining salt is hidden in processed and quick-service foods. Think about this: almost ¾ teaspoon of added salt is necessary to equal the sodium content in just three pieces of Kentucky Fried Chicken (1,396 mg). Just such a fact convinces me that we must return in large part to the diet of days past—to whole grains, legumes (dried beans and peas), fresh vegetables and fruits, and, for those who choose them, certain meats and fish. Most of these foods are extremely low in sodium.

Try decreasing your salt intake gradually. One way is to utilize food charts and choose low-salt alternatives. Many people find help in some of the excellent books that have been published over the past decade. Some of these are

1. Ralph E. Minear, M.D. *The Joy of Living Salt-Free.* New York: Macmillan, 1984.
2. Craig Claiborne. *Craig Claiborne's Gourmet Diet.* New York: Ballantine, 1980.
3. Jane Brody. *Jane Brody's Good Food Cookbook.* New York: Norton, 1986.

4. Harriet Roth. *Deliciously Low: The Gourmet Guide to Low-Sodium, Low-Cholesterol, and Low-Sugar Cooking.* New York: New American Library, 1983.
5. Michael Jacobson, Bonnie F. Liebman, and Greg Moyer. *Salt: The Brand Name Diet to Sodium Contents.* Washington, D.C.: Center for Science in the Public Interest, 1983.

Another good way to learn to live with less salt is to learn how to season food with herbs and spices. Examples of seasonings to try on various foods are listed in table 14. Although you may not believe it now, with well-prepared foods, it is usually difficult to tell whether salt or some other seasoning has been used as flavoring.

Table 14

Seasonings to Use Instead of Salt

MEAT, FISH, AND POULTRY

Beef	Bay leaf, dry mustard powder, green pepper, marjoram, fresh mushrooms, nutmeg, onion, pepper, sage, thyme
Chicken	Green pepper, lemon juice, marjoram, fresh mushrooms, paprika, parsley, poultry seasoning, sage, thyme
Fish	Bay leaf, curry powder, dry mustard, green pepper, lemon juice, marjoram, fresh mushrooms, paprika
Lamb	Curry powder, garlic, mint, mint jelly, pineapple, rosemary
Pork	Apple, applesauce, garlic, onion, sage
Veal	Apricot, bay leaf, curry powder, ginger, marjoram, oregano

VEGETABLES

Asparagus	Garlic, lemon juice, onion, vinegar
Corn	Green pepper, pimiento, fresh tomato
Cucumbers	Chives, dill, garlic, vinegar
Green beans	Dill, lemon juice, marjoram, nutmeg, pimiento
Greens	Onion, pepper, vinegar
Peas	Green pepper, mint, fresh mushrooms, onion, parsley
Potatoes	Green pepper, mace, onion, paprika, parsley
Rice	Chives, green pepper, onion, pimiento, saffron
Squash	Brown sugar, cinnamon, ginger, mace, nutmeg, onion
Tomatoes	Basil, marjoram, onion, oregano

SOUPS

Bean	Dry mustard (pinch)
Milk chowders	Peppercorns
Pea	Bay leaf, parsley
Vegetable	Vinegar, red or white pepper, chives, parsley

Source: Cooking Without Your Salt Shaker *(New York: American Heart Association, 1978).*

People starting to lower their salt intake often ask questions about salt substitutes and sea salt. At the present, there are about fourteen salt substitutes on the market. Potassium chloride rather than sodium chloride is their primary ingredient. The most popular ones are No Salt, Morton's Salt Substitute, and Adolph's Salt Substitute.

The safety of these potassium substances is controversial because of the danger of consuming excess potassium, which can cause heart and kidney problems. However, under a physician's guidance (where the blood potassium level can be monitored if necessary), use of salt substitutes in moderate amounts should be no problem and can help you limit your sodium intake.

Natural food proponents consider sea salt to be a better kind of salt because it has more minerals. However, many observers assert that the majority of the minerals are removed during processing, which means that sea salt is no better than regular salt and is much more expensive.

Dr. Jimmy Scott says some commercial products similar to sea salt still contain trace minerals and an excellent balance of sodium to potassium.[1] He suggests that people who desire a salty taste use Wachter's Sea-Land Seasoning. This is a mixture of sea vegetation and vegetables.

Finally, the long-held belief about hot weather, sweating, and salt tablets bears discussion. "Doc, I sweat a lot on my job, so don't I need extra salt?" I have heard this often, but the truth is that people seldom become salt-depleted by sweating. Only if you lose more than three quarts of fluid and lose six pounds in a single day will you probably need to add some salt to your diet. The amount is best figured by allowing an additional ⅓ to 1 teaspoon of salt for each quart of water (above the three quarts) you lose. Thus, August athletes, summer construction workers, and workers in hot, closed spaces do sometimes need to be aware of the possibility of salt depletion. In my twenty years as a physician, however, I have seen only two people with salt depletion from sweating. In those same twenty years, I have seen thousands of people with some sort of medical problem related at least in part to excess salt intake. The important point to remember if you sweat a lot is to drink more water, enough so you don't become thirsty. Thirst indicates dehydration.

Changing your salt intake can make a difference in how you feel. Go ahead, give it a try!

Notes

1. J. Scott, "How Salt Affects Your Health," *International Journal of Holistic Health and Medicine* (Summer 1985): 20.

III

Sugar—Is It All That Nice?

Do you have any of these problems?

Abdominal pains
Allergies
Anxiety
Bed-wetting
Bloating
Breast tenderness
Cravings for sweets
Dental cavities
Depression and crying bouts
Diabetes mellitus
Diarrhea
Dizziness and vertigo
Excessive flu, colds, or
  infection
Excessive sweating
Fainting
Fatigue, lethargy, exhaustion
Flatulence
Gum disease (gingivitis)
Headaches
Heart disease
High cholesterol level
High triglyceride level
Hives
Hyperactivity
Hypoglycemia
Insomnia
Irritability
Irritable colon
Itching
Kidney stones
Memory loss
Menstrual pain
Moodiness and mood
  swings
Muscle aches
Nausea
Obesity
Osteoporosis
Polysystemic chronic
  candidiasis
Poor concentration
Premenstrual syndrome
Seizures
Skin nodules
Skin rashes
Speedy heart rate
Swollen voice box (laryngeal
  edema)
Tremors
Vaginal discharge
Vaginal itching
Vaginitis
Weakness
Yeast infection

If you are bothered by any of these problems, you may be experiencing the side effects of sugar or other sweeteners.

Chapter 6

The Real Problems Sugar Causes

Controversy surrounds all aspects of diet and health, but sugar leads the way in terms of divergent opinions. Some articles say that diabetes (hyperglycemia or high blood sugar) is ten times more common than hypoglycemia (low blood sugar). Other reports say that hypoglycemia is ten times more common than diabetes. No wonder people are confused!

Does sugar cause hyperactivity in children? Many parents and a few scientists say *yes!* Most medical doctors say *no!* How about mood swings? PMS? Fatigue?

About the only health problem for which a connection to sugar is agreed upon is dental cavities. And even here, argument exists over the effect of the amount of sugar eaten versus when it is eaten (with or between meals) versus the *type* of sugar that is eaten (sticky or smooth). The data form a confusing hodgepodge to anyone trying to discover the truth. Let's take a look at some of the problems and diseases that are possibly related to sugar consumption.

Fatigue

Ted came to me quite sure he had a serious illness. For four to six months, this dynamic 38-year-old businessman had been tired, lacked energy, and been unable to complete some of his business projects. He had been divorced twelve months previously but said he was over that ordeal and involved in a new relationship.

Ted had really changed his eating pattern over the past year. Since no one made his breakfast for him each morning, he had simply quit eating it. Instead, he grabbed a sweet roll or doughnut at midmorning. At lunch he ate out with clients, usually choosing the restaurant "special." For supper, he stopped for fast food such as a hamburger, fries, and a malt. He drank two to three cans of Pepsi-Cola daily and frequently snacked on candy bars or cookies.

Clearly, Ted was eating no whole grains or fruits, and he had a vegetable only rarely. His sugar intake was very high. I asked Ted if he would be willing to try some radical dietary changes for just two weeks. He said he would do anything, because his business was going to fall apart if he didn't pep up very quickly.

He began to eat a whole-grain cereal, whole-wheat toast, and fruit each morning. At lunch he had a salad, soup, raw vegetables, or a vegetable or tuna sandwich plus fruit. His evening meals were stir-fry vegetables, brown rice, whole-grain spaghetti with tofu or ground beef, various vegetables and pasta dishes, and a couple of fish or lean-meat meals with a potato and vegetable. For snacks, he had low-fat cheese, fresh or dried fruit, and raw vegetables. For a beverage he drank water.

Ted was slated to return to me in two weeks. On the eleventh day, Ted stormed into my office saying he was cancelling his follow-up appointment. He felt better than he had in five years! He told me that his energy level was great and that he had already finished a major paper he had been trying to write for two months.

You can see why it would be difficult to convince Ted—or me—that sugar intake is not a significant contributor to fatigue and low energy.

Dental Cavities

Some years ago, Joey, age 4, had recurrent ear infections, so I prescribed medicine for three months of the winter. He took an antibiotic (Gantrisin) twice daily, plus a decongestant (Actifed) three times daily. The next summer, Joey saw his dentist and had fourteen cavities. I later realized that from January to March, five times each day, Joey had been drinking a sticky, sugary syrup—the medicine I had prescribed for him. Gantrisin and Actifed, as well as many pediatric suspension drugs, are 50 percent to 70 percent sugar. I learned a very important lesson about liquid medications and what sticky, sugary substances can do to teeth.

Most researchers agree that sugar consumption correlates with dental cavities and gum disease (gingivitis). But has the public responded to this widely disseminated information by eating less sugar? No. Instead, we put a chemical (fluoride) in the water to counteract the negative effect of the sugar intake. No one will deny that fluoride works to help prevent dental cavities. The problem is that fluoride does not help prevent the numerous other health problems to which sugar contributes.

I consider dental cavities a wonderful signal that we need to decrease our sugar intake. When we block that signal by means of fluoride and fail to decrease sugar intake, we then go on to develop many of the problems and diseases described in this chapter. Sugar needs to be a twice-a-week treat, not a twice-a-day treatment for loneliness, fatigue, food cravings, or sadness!

Heart Disease

The connection between sugar and cavities is easy to understand. But what about sugar and heart disease? This relationship is a bit more complicated. Increased sugar intake causes the body to produce more insulin, which helps in sugar digestion. Insulin then directs the conversion of sugar into fatty acids and triglycerides, which cause hardening of the arteries, a condition that can lead to heart attacks.

Some studies have demonstrated that people on a high-sugar

diet develop much higher levels of fats in their blood than people on a low-sugar diet.[1] A study of people in Norway during World War II showed a marked decrease in the number of deaths from heart disease during the war years, a time when the consumption of sugar and fat was much lower than usual.[2]

Obesity and Diabetes

One thing that makes a person overweight is eating more calories than the body uses up. Eating sugary foods is a very easy way of taking in excessive calories, since a lot of sugar calories can be packed into a very small quantity of food. Also, eating sweets does not tend to fill you up, so you eat excess calories. For example, one pound of apples contains 260 calories, while one pound of Baby Ruth candy bars has about 2,300 calories—nine times more calories in the same quantity of food! Also, the apples contain no fat, but the candy bars contain 96 gm (19 teaspoons) of fat!

Obviously, it's easy to gain weight if you eat sweets. Since excess weight in adults is very closely connected to the risk of diabetes mellitus (non-insulin-dependent type*), it is quite possible that a connection exists between high sugar intake and diabetes. In fact, one study showed that a diet of simple carbohydrates, such as sugars and processed foods, caused subjects to exhibit specific diabetic symptoms.[3] Remember, a family history of diabetes does not mean you will get diabetes. By changing your diet, you can improve your chances of avoiding the disease radically.

There are two types of diabetes. Type I is called the insulin-dependent type, because its treatment usually includes insulin shots. Type II is called the non-insulin-dependent type, because its treatment requires weight loss and diet modification but usually not insulin. About 90 percent of diabetics have Type II.

Osteoporosis

The connection of osteoporosis, or bone loss, and excess sugar intake is more controversial. We know that excesss dietary sugar causes increased copper loss in the urine. Decreased copper levels in the body can have an adverse effect on bone mineralization, since bones need such minerals as copper and zinc as well as calcium for strength. Highly sugared soft drinks have a high phosphorus (13 mg/oz.), low calcium (0 mg/oz.) ratio. This imbalance between phosphorus and calcium encourages hyperparathyroidism and subsequent bone loss.[4]

Reactive Hypoglycemia

As noted earlier, the opposite of diabetes (high blood sugar or *hyper*glycemia) is low blood sugar (*hypo*glycemia). In 1949, Dr. Seale Harris was awarded the American Medical Association (AMA) Distinguished Service Medal for Research that led to the discovery of hypoglycemia. Yet in 1973, the AMA basically labeled most reactive hypoglycemia a "nondisease." The association stated that the hypoglycemia patient's problems were primarily psychological in origin. In other words, most hypoglycemic patients were simply neurotic. This conclusion caused quite a furor, as you might have suspected, because many patients and physicians disagreed with it. Thousands of hypoglycemic patients had tried years of psychotherapy with minimal improvement in their mood swings, depression, fatigue, irritability, poor memory, and lightheadedness. Then, when treated nutritionally with a diet high in complex carbohydrates or protein and low in the simple carbohydrates such as white sugar and white flour, they improved dramatically. It is very difficult to convince those people that their problem was mainly psychological.

The determining factor behind the AMA's hypoglycemia edict was the unreliability of the one test used to diagnose reactive hypoglycemia (the six-hour glucose tolerance test). Some normal people will have no symptoms when their blood sugar level is less than 50 mg (supposedly the cutoff point to diagnose hypoglycemia), while many hypoglycemics get dizzy, headachy, weak, and sleepy with a blood sugar level of 75 mg. Some researchers believe we need to measure other parameters besides blood sugar level to determine whether hypoglycemia exists in a patient. Such studies as brain wave activity,[5] glucagon levels,[6] and adrenalin levels may give a much more accurate indication.

Strangely enough, we in medicine, for all our insistence on empiricism, at times maintain a double standard. We accept the fact that some *hyper*glycemic patients (diabetics) have blood sugar levels of 400 mg with no symptoms, while others have multiple symptoms when their blood sugar is running only 300 mg. But, unaccountably, we are not as accepting of the fact that *low* blood sugar levels affect different people differently.

We find another example of individual physiologic variability with respect to blood pressure readings. Many of my patients feel no differently whether their blood pressure is 130 or 230 mm HG. Others notice a number of symptoms, such as weakness, tiredness, or headaches, with only a slight blood pressure elevation to 160 or 170. Doesn't it seem peculiar that we accept *these* variations as being normal but consider the variations in symptoms related to differing levels of blood sugar to be neurotic? The two basic dietary causes of hypoglycemic problems are excess sugars or processed foods in our diets and excess dietary fats.[7] Both factors cause abnormal sugar fluctuations (reactive hypoglycemia) in many people.

Some of the symptoms attributable to reactive hypoglycemia are

- anxiety
- craving for sweets
- depression and crying bouts

- dizziness and vertigo
- fainting
- fast heart rate
- fatigue, lethargy, and exhaustion
- headaches
- heart palpitations
- insomnia
- irritability
- moodiness and mood swings
- poor concentration
- poor memory
- sweating
- tremors
- weakness

Some or all of these symptoms can, of course, accompany depressions and/or anxiety. But in many cases, all it takes to relieve the symptoms is a simple change in diet. For most people with these symptoms, a fourteen-day sugar-elimination trial is well worth the effort.

A popular book telling most of what you need to know about hypoglycemia is Dr. Paavo Airola's *Hypoglycemia: A Better Approach*.[8] In general, I agree with what Dr. Airola says, but I disagree with his recommendation that a patient undergo a six-hour oral glucose tolerance test to diagnose hypoglycemia. The test itself is expensive and time consuming, and many hypoglycemic patients become quite ill during the testing. I have found that taking a thorough history plus a review of a trial of dietary change are usually sufficient for diagnosis.

Interestingly, Dr. Airola's suggested diet for hypoglycemia is very similar to the low-fat, high-fiber diet recommended by Nathan Pritikin and John McDougall, which I discuss in chapters 10 and 11. Whole grains, legumes, vegetables, and fruits are what Dr. Airola calls "the optimum diet." He also adds seeds and nuts to that diet. Remember, this was the primary diet of most of our ancestors for thousands of years.

The high-protein diet recommended by some doctors for hypoglycemia will give temporary help to many people. Unfortunately, use of this diet over a long period of time will often increase a person's risk for heart disease, cancer, and other degenerative diseases. Remember, high protein generally means high fat intake. I recommend a high-protein diet for any problem only rarely.

In my experience, 80 percent to 90 percent of people who return to the more natural diet of our ancestors feel better, have more energy, and become ill less frequently. Few pills or surgical procedures come close to producing those kinds of results.

Vaginal Yeast Infections

Betty came to see me quite frustrated. She was twenty-five years old and had been treated about ten times over the past four years for vaginal yeast infections. She had tried many creams, foams, and suppositories and had even tried long periods of abstinence from sexual intercourse. She had also tried douching, wearing underclothing of different materials, and stopping the use of tampons. All her efforts seemed to be of no use. She continued to experience bouts of vaginal itching, burning, and discharge.

Betty is an excellent example of a person with a very common problem that is often solved by a simple dietary change. Upon questioning Betty, I found that her diet was quite high in sugar. When I suggested a low-sugar diet, Betty said she was willing to try anything. Her problem was driving her crazy.

Betty began to follow my suggestions for dietary changes carefully. She was amazed to find that after one more bout of itching and discharge, she remained free of yeast problems at one- and two-year follow-up visits.

I was not surprised. Numerous women had responded similarly. A 1984 study showed that if women with recurrent vaginal yeast infections decreased sucrose and milk sugars in their
diets, 80 percent would not have a yeast infection during the
following year.[9]

Premenstrual Syndrome (PMS) and Polysystemic Chronic Candidiasis (PCC or Chronic Yeast)

These two controversial problems have received tremendous
publicity in the 1980s. PMS is the presence of specific symptoms during the week or two prior to menstruation. Following menstruation, there is a symptom-free week. The most
common of the more than one hundred possible symptoms are
irritability, mood swings, bloating, fatigue, food cravings,
depression, and breast tenderness. The cyclical nature of the
symptoms is the key to diagnosis.

Polysystemic chronic candidiasis (PCC) is also the presence
of a group of specific symptoms, but these are not due to hormonal changes as is PMS. The symptoms of PCC are thought
to result from toxins produced by the uncontrolled growth of
the usually benign yeast called *Candida albicans*. The over-
whelming yeast growth is thought to result from a number of
insults to the body that lower the immune system's ability to
fight off problems. Such insults include antibiotics, birth control pills, cortisone, stress, environmental toxins, allergies, and
nutritional deficiencies resulting from excess intake of sugar
and processed foods. Major symptoms include all of those listed
for PMS, plus weakness, muscle or joint soreness, and "feeling sick all over."

You can see why patients with PMS or PCC are considered
hypochondriacal or neurotic by the majority of physicians. The
symptoms are vague and nonspecific. There is no good blood

test yet developed that could easily confirm the diagnosis. There are no good studies proving that treatment works. Interestingly, we physicians commonly diagnose influenza and multiple sclerosis (MS), which are also complex problems associated with multiple vague symptoms and complaints. And with these conditions, a blood test will not give the diagnosis and there are no good studies proving the effectiveness of treatment.

I find it hard to understand why physicians are wary of diagnosing and treating PMS or PCC. In most people, an essential part of treating these conditions is dietary change, which on a trial basis can't hurt anyone. There are thousands of people who feel quite strongly that dietary treatment for PMS or PCC completely changed their life. Most of these people had seen numerous physicians and counselors previously without good results.

In my experience, the majority of patients suffering from PMS and PCC improve markedly when they make certain dietary changes. The two biggest changes are avoidance of most simple carbohydrates (the sugars and processed grains) and an increased intake of roughage and fiber (whole grains, vegetables, legumes, and fruits).

I believe that sugar intake plays a significant role in both of these problems. For readers interested in more details about PMS, I recommend an excellent two-part article by Kaaren Nichols, M.D., in the March 1986 and July 1986 issues of *Holistic Medicine*. The first part gives the details regarding the possible causes and treatment of PMS. The second provocatively explores the possibility that PMS is a myth imposed on women. Nichols states that the two premenstrual weeks are really a time of strength, creativity, and assertive energy. She adds that it is time for women to be less passive and submissive than our society now wants them to be. She concludes that premenstrual changes can, instead of causing a diseased and dreadful time, help women tap into their own unique qualities, strengths, and energies.

For more information on chronic yeast problems, check these three excellent sources:

1. Christianne Northrup, M.D. "Freedom from Yeast Infections," *East West Journal* (July 1986).
2. William G. Crook. *The Yeast Connection.* Jackson, Tenn.: Professional Books, 1986. Order from the publisher at P.O. Box 3494, Jackson, TN 38301.
3. John Trowbridge, M.D. *The Yeast Syndrome.* New York: Bantam, 1986.

Bed-Wetting (Enuresis)

Jane was a 7-year-old who refused to stay overnight with grandparents or girlfriends. Why? Because she wet the bed every night. But on the fourth night of a two-week sugar-elimination diet, Jane did not wet the bed, nor did she ever again unless she ate some sugar products.

Medical science says that food allergies rarely if ever cause bed-wetting. In my experience, and in the experience of some other physicians, food allergy is a rather common cause of bed-wetting.[10] The most common offenders I have found are citrus (usually excessive amounts of orange juice), apple juice, milk, tomatoes, food colorings, and corn. You are undoubtedly wondering how these foods and substances relate to sugar. Up to 50 percent of the foods we eat with sugar in them are made with corn syrup, as are the majority of soft drinks. So a 7-year-old may have a rather large corn intake that is a hidden cause of allergic bed-wetting.

Poor Exercise Endurance

For years we have heard tales about trainers giving athletes candy or soda pop during exercise to improve their performance.

"Sugar will give quick energy," state ads from the sugar industry. The claim is accurate as far as it goes, but unfortunately, it does not mention that the quick energy lasts only minutes. Insulin pours out in response to ingested sugar, and soon afterwards our blood sugar level is back to normal or may be even *lower* than it was initially.

A recent study of five athletes showed that drinking a 12-ounce sugar drink (one can of pop) one hour before exercise decreased endurance by 25 percent.*[11] In other words, an athlete so affected would be able to run a 6-minute mile instead of a 4.5-minute mile. The findings of this study are quite dramatic, but I have not been able to find any other study relating sugar intake and exercise endurance. That seems most unusual to me, considering America's passion for sports.

Like most rules, this one has exceptions. In rare cases, sugar may benefit some athletes. For instance, marathoners running on a cold day (when water loss is minimal) have found that some sugar intake during the run may be beneficial.[12] But as a general rule, the less sugar and simple carbohydrates all of us (including athletes) eat, the better off we will be.

Increased Incidence of Infections

Do you get more flus or colds than you believe you should? Do your kids have frequent bouts of ear infection or tonsillitis? You may be correct in thinking that it is just not right to "pick up every darn bug that comes along!"

Well, the cause may simply be excess dietary sugar! Before you write this statement off as foolish, I would like you to

* *The sugar causes insulin to be released for digestion. Since a processed food such as sugar is already partially "broken down," digestion takes place quickly. The excess insulin then digests more blood sugar—the reservoir. This process is experienced as a quick "high" but also a quick drop-off—or decreased endurance.*

consider three points:

1. Do you recall as a child being ill as often as your kids
   are now? Were your parents sick as often as you are now
   sick? The answer is usually no for both these questions.
2. When a virus is "going around," why do some people get
   bad cases, others mild cases, and still others no illness
   at all? Is it germs that cause the flu problems or is it
   our immune system's inability to fight off the invading
   germs?
3. Many studies show that sugar and other simple carbohydrates cause a reduction in our body's defense against
   such invaders as bacteria and viruses.[13]

One theory suggests that the reason we get more colds and
infections than our parents did and that our children get more
than we did as children is that our sugar consumption has
increased fourfold in the past 100 years. This increase has
reduced the ability of our immune systems to fight infection.
This may be why new infectious diseases seem to be appearing every few years—Legionnaires' disease, toxic shock syndrome, and now AIDS, the most devastating immune system
disease yet.

Unfortunately, we have made Louis Pasteur's wonderful discovery of the "germ theory" *the* answer to infections. As a
nation, we prefer to believe that the illnesses we suffer from
are the result of external forces alone. In reality, illnesses are
the result of many variables. Rather than focusing so much on
the "germ," maybe it is time to begin to improve those aspects
of our lives that weaken our immune systems and predispose
us to illnesses and diseases. The primary areas needing evaluation in our lives are the spiritual, social, mental, emotional,
and physical aspects. We can usually effect a major improvement in our physical lives by eating foods that are nourishing,
wholesome, and truly from the earth. Processed foods do not
fulfill these criteria!

So, before blaming the Chinese for the "Hong Kong flu" or animals for "swine flu," let us focus more on ourselves—on conditions in our lives that may be predisposing us to infection from those microorganisms.

Kidney Stones

Kidney stones are not a well known side effect of sugar consumption, but they are one that "stone sufferers" should know about. A British study in 1986 revealed a link between sugar consumption and increased calcium oxalate (the crystals in the majority of stones) in the urine.[14]

Isn't it fascinating that even kidney stones could be related to excess sugar in the diet? Likewise, dental cavities at a young age might be considered warnings against excess sugar consumption. It could be that we are actually unlucky that fluoride works so well in eliminating cavities, because it masks the underlying problem.

Hyperactivity and Mood Swings

Last but certainly not least in controversy is the relationship between sugar intake and hyperactivity, "acting out," and mood swings. Suzy was six years old when her parents found a note from her saying that she had run away from home. For the previous six to eight months she had been having extreme mood swings. "One day she's a neat, lovable child," her mother told me, "but the next day she'll be very hyper, belligerent, and anxious. She'll jump from one thing to another." When we put Suzy on a sugar-elimination diet, she began to have only good days. If she ate some sweets, the hyperactivity and mood swings would quickly begin again. Physicians will have a difficult time convincing Suzy's mom and dad that her problems are not sugar related. Eating sugar literally "turns her on like a switch," and she is just fine when she is off sugar.

I am not sure why researchers studying hyperactivity and sugar have come up with such diverse findings, but Dr. C. Keith Connors gives some reasons. He believes the researchers use samples that are too small and have age ranges that are too wide, that they use insensitive measures of testing, and that they often ignore what else, besides sugar, the child is eating. Dr. Connors's own study found a clear linear relationship between increased sugar intake and deviant behavior.[15] Interestingly, if the children in Connors's study ate a good breakfast with enough protein, excess sugar did not seem to bother them.

Dr. Connors's study is not an isolated example. Multiple researchers have found close links between dietary sugar and hyperactivity and deviant behavior problems.[16] Other studies, however, show no link between diet and behavior. To me, finding out whether our children or we ourselves are intolerant of dietary sugars seems critically important. I believe we ought to be willing to spend millions of research dollars to answer this question. Instead, our industries spend millions of dollars researching and selling various drugs to suppress hyperactivity. To me this is evidence of mistaken priorities.

You can now begin to see why I believe sugar in our diet causes many symptoms and diseases. It is difficult to understand why medical authorities continue to argue so vociferously in favor of eating sugar. It reminds me of how we physicians handled alcohol problems in the 1960s. The only people we called alcoholics then were Skid Row bums and a few of our patients with cirrhosis. But the 1970s revealed that there were 10 to 20 million alcoholics in the United States and that many of them were physicians!

I believe the same problem is now occurring with regard to "sugaraholics" within the medical profession. If we admit that sugar causes health problems, we doctors will have to look at our own sugar consumption, and we just do not want to do that.

Can sugar really be as addictive as alcohol? Let's explore that further in chapter 7.

Notes

1. J. Yudkin, *Sweet and Dangerous* (New York: Bantam Books, 1972).
2. A. Strom, "Mortality from Circulatory Diseases in Norway, 1940–45," *Lancet* 1 (1951): 126.
3. A. M. Cohen et al., "Effect of Interchanging Bread and Sugar as Main Source of Carbohydrate on Glucose Tolerance," *American Journal of Clinical Nutrition* (1966): 59.
4. J. Bland, "Calcium Pushers," *East West Journal* 17 (1987): 70.
5. W. J. Hudspeth et al., "Neurobiology of the Hypoglycemia Syndrome," *Journal of Holistic Medicine* 3 (1981): 60–71.
6. P. F. Piero et al., "Reactive Hypoglycemia and A-cell Glucagon Deficiency in the Adult," *Journal of the American Medical Association* 24 (1980): 2281.
7. G. Haber et al., "Depletion and Disruption of Dietary Fiber," *Lancet* 2 (1977): 679; and J. Olefsky et al., "Reappraisal of the Role of Insulin in Hypertriglyceridemia," *American Journal of Medicine* 57 (1974): 551
8. P. Airola, *Hypoglycemia: A Better Approach* (Phoenix, Ariz.: Health Plus, 1977).
9. B. J. Horowitz et al., "Sugar Chromatography and Recurrent Candida Vulvovaginitis," *Journal of Reproductive Medicine* 29 (1984): 441.
10. F. Speer, "What to Do About Food Allergies?" *Consultant* (October 1973): 142.
11. K. Keller and R. Schwarzkoph, "Pre-Exercise Snacks May Decrease Exercise Performance," *Physician and Sports Medicine* 12 (1984): 89.
12. Ibid.
13. W. M. Ringsdorf et al., "Sucrose, Neutrophilic Phagocytosis and Resistance to Disease," *Dental Survey* (December 1976): 46–48; A. Sanchez et al., "Role of Sugar in Human Neutrophilic Phagocytosis," *American Journal of Clinical Nutrition* 26 (November 1973): 1180; and E. Kijak et al., "Relationship of Blood Sugar Level and Leukocytic Phagocytosis," *Journal of Southern California State Dental Associates* 32 (1964): 349.

14. M. K. Li et al., "Does Sucrose Damage Kidneys?" *British Journal of Urology* 58 (August 1986): 353–57.
15. C. Connors, "Moderate Amount of Sugar Seems to Aid Classroom Performance," *Family Practice News* 15 (1985): 71.
16. L. Langseth and J. Dowd, "Glucose Tolerance and Hyperkinesis," *Food, Cosmetology, Toxicology* 16 (1979): 129; A. J. Lewis, "The Junk Food Made Me Do It," *East West Journal* 15 (1985): 66; A. Schauss, "Dietary Intervention Improves Delinquent Behavior," *Price-Pottenger Nutrition Foundation Journal* 10 (1986): 14; and H. W. Powers, "Dietary Measures to Improve Behavior and Achievement," *Academic Therapy* IX (1973–1974): 203–15.

Chapter 7

Sugar Is Everywhere

"If you clean your plate, you can have dessert!"
"If I finish this job quickly, I'll treat myself to a piece of pie."
"I love to go trick-or-treating on Halloween and splurge on the candy along with the kids."
"Well, since I did aerobics for an hour, I guess I can have some ice cream."
When the dessert tray is brought to the restaurant table, notice the nervous laughter and numerous self-conscious comments it evokes. We Americans seem to have an obsessional love-hate relationship with sugar. We think and talk about avoiding it but are continually "giving in" to be sociable, to reward ourselves, or just because we can't stand to go without it. Does this behavior remind you of the behavior surrounding the use of any other type of substances? How about alcohol? Nicotine? Coffee? Yes, sugar ranks with these other legal and acceptable addictions. I say *addictions* because it is very easy to substitute the word *sugar* when listing the criteria with which we diagnose an alcohol or drug addiction.

Figure 1 is an example of a typical questionnaire used to help people decide if they are alcoholics. I have made only one change in it: to substitute *sugar* for *alcohol*. Test yourself using figure 1 to see if you might be a sugaraholic. One *yes* answer in this test is a definite warning that you may be a sugaraholic. Two indicate you probably *are* a sugaraholic. Checking *yes* three or more times definitely indicates sugaraholism.

Does it seem a bit strange to you to compare alcohol addiction with sugar problems? I hope after reading in the preceding chapter of the tremendous number of diseases to which sugar might contribute, such a comparison begins to make

Figure 1

Are You a Sugaraholic?

	Yes	No
Do you lose time at work because of eating sugar snacks?	___	___
Does excess sugar eating ever make your home life unhappy or cause arguments?	___	___
Have you ever felt remorse after eating sugar foods?	___	___
Has your energy or ambition decreased since eating more sugar foods?	___	___
Do you crave sugar or chocolate at a definite time of day?	___	___
Does eating sugar foods ever cause you to have difficulty sleeping?	___	___
Has your efficiency decreased since eating more sugar foods?	___	___
Do you eat sugar foods to escape from worries or troubles?	___	___
Do you eat sugar foods alone?	___	___
Has your physician or dentist ever treated you for any problems possibly related to sugar consumption?	___	___

sense to you. Alcoholics often have trouble stopping the use of alcohol even when they are aware that it causes health problems. Now think of the people you know who have weight problems, diabetes, hypertension, recurrent flu, or a lack of energy and still are unable or unwilling to avoid sugar foods.

For years, comedians and, in fact, all of us joked about alcohol problems and alcoholics. In learning more about alcohol, however, we came to realize that alcoholism is not a joking matter. We have not yet learned the same lesson about sugar. That is why we still hear nervous laughter and jokes when the dessert tray appears at a restaurant.

Why Do We Crave Sugar?

Sugar-rich foods are universally accepted by most humans in preference to other foods. This response to sweet taste may be the result of millions of years of food-selection habits. Dr. Jeffrey Bland suggests that our foraging hunter-gatherer ancestors recognized a sweet taste as a signal that the food bearing it could provide calories for energy.[1] Most forage has a high cellulose concentration, has no apparent taste, and, because it is indigestible, gives humans no nutrients. The assumption is, therefore, that a sweet taste would have directed our ancestors to the foods containing calories and nutrients.

Only in the last century have we begun to concentrate sweetness in foods and produce high-sugar foods. So, as with many other things in life, what was once advantageous and helpful has become detrimental to our health and our lives. We need to retrain the satiety and hunger centers in our brains to respond properly to a diet of diverse, nonsweetened foods.

Let's take a look, in Figure 2 and Table 15, at the two sources of sugar, sugar cane and sugar beets, to see what happens to these wonderful, natural foods after we process them. Can you believe the nutritional differences between white sugar and molasses, as revealed by the table? These results show quite dramatically the effects of processing and changing foods. Both sugar cane and sugar beets are extremely healthy foods, loaded

with nutrients. Yet the white sugar that results after processing is basically a nonfood. It contains no fiber, no vitamins,
and almost no minerals. For this reason, we call sugar foods
"empty calories," or junk food.

What's Wrong with Empty Calories?

Since sugar contains almost no nutritional value, people for
whom 25 percent of their total calories are sugar (a common
percentage) need to obtain 100 percent of their nutrients (vitamins and minerals) from 75 percent of their total calories. Some
children even eat 50 percent of their total calories in sugar,
meaning that they must consume all their nutrients in just
50 percent of their food. This gives you a good idea of why we
Americans often fail to get adequate nutrients in our diet. As
an example, in 1987 I did a computerized nutritional analysis
on fifty patients who were coming to see me at the Wellness
Center of Minnesota in Mankato. The results showed that not
one of these patients was receiving the recommended daily
allowance (RDA) of the fourteen vitamins and minerals evalu-

Figure 2

Where Does Sugar Come From?

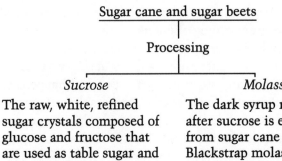

Sugar cane and sugar beets

Processing

Sucrose	*Molasses*
The raw, white, refined sugar crystals composed of glucose and fructose that are used as table sugar and are added to many foods and food products.	The dark syrup remaining after sucrose is extracted from sugar cane and beets. Blackstrap molasses is the concentrated syrup remaining after three extractions.

ated. Many of the people analyzed were failing to receive the RDA of the majority of vitamins and minerals, and only three of the fifty were deficient in only one vitamin or one mineral. Nevertheless, many of these people thought they were eating extremely healthy diets based on the four food groups and were amazed at the results of my analyses.

Besides displacing essential nutrients in the diet, sugar robs stored vitamins and minerals from the body. The conversion of sugars into energy requires vitamins and minerals. So sugars enter our bodies as empty calories and then force our bodies to use their own nutrients for digestion. This should begin to suggest to you why excess sugar consumption is not a healthy habit.

If we take in 45 percent of our calories as fat calories and 25 percent as sugar foods, that means 70 percent of our intake contains little or no fiber and roughage. Is it any wonder that we are such a constipated nation? The question certainly bears asking here, though I will explore the issue in detail in a later chapter.

Table 15

Nutrient Content of Sugar

	1 cup white sugar (sucrose)	1 cup blackstrap molasses (mg)
Calcium	0	2,192
Phosphorus	0	272
Iron	0.2	51
Potassium	6.0	9,360
Thiamin (B₁)	0	0.32
Riboflavin (B₂)	0	0.64
Niacin (B₃)	0	6.4

Source: S. R. Williams, Nutrition and Diet Therapy (St. Louis: Times Mirror/Mosby, 1985), Appendix A26. Reproduced by permission from S. R. Williams, Nutrition and Diet Therapy (St. Louis: The C. V. Mosby Co., 1985).

Why Our Forbears Seemed Unaffected

Various figures are available, but most observers will agree that American sugar consumption has risen dramatically over the last sixty to one hundred years. The figures vary in accordance with what is being measured, whether sucrose only (table sugar) or all processed sugars (such as corn sweeteners, molasses, lactose, and honey). In general, a consensus estimate is that sugar consumption has risen from approximately 30 or 40 pounds per person per year in 1880 to 130 pounds per person in 1980.[2] You know what a one-pound box of sugar looks like. Each of us, on average, consumes the equivalent of more than two of these boxes every week!

Despite the fact that our recent ancestors undoubtedly ate dessert quite often and consumed cookies and cake at snack time, their hidden sugar intake was very low. We tend to believe our grandparents ate more sugar than we do. The reason for this misconception is that in the early 1900s, 75 percent of all the sugar consumed was added to foods at home during baking or at the table. You could *see* what you were eating. Now 75 percent of the sugar we consume is "hidden" in the processed foods we buy at the store, and only 25 percent is added directly at home.[3] In this, as you will recall, sugar bears a similarity to salt.

Many of my patients are like Henry, a man in his twenties. He said he rarely if ever ate sweets or sugar foods. On further questioning, though, he told me that he drank six cans of Dr. Pepper daily. He was consuming the equivalent of seventy-two teaspoons of sugar each day!

Sugar is hidden in most cereals, yogurts, ketchups, salad dressings, soups, vitamins, and even medications. Do you remember my story about 5-year-old Joey and his cavities? His tooth problem was medicine-related because he took medicine with lots of sugar all winter long. See table 16 for an overview of sugary medications.

Table 16

The Sugar Content of Commonly Prescribed Liquid Medications

Medication	gm/5ml	%	Sugar form
Actifed, syrup	3.50	70	Sucrose
Chlor-Trimeton, expectorant	3.00	60	Sucrose
Compazine, syrup	3.50	70	Sucrose
Dexedrine, elixir	0.75	15	Sucrose
Dilantin-30, suspension	1.04	21	Sucrose
Dimetapp, elixir	0	0	
Gantrisin, suspension I	2.77	55	Sucrose
Gantrisin, syrup	3.50	70	Sucrose
Ilosone, liquid	2.00	40	Sucrose
Lanoxin, elixir	1.50	30	Sucrose
Phenobarbital, elixir	0.64	13	Sucrose
Robitussin, syrup	2.80	15	Glucose/fructose
Rondec, DM, syrup	3.70	74	Glucose/fructose
Sudafed, syrup	3.50	70	Sucrose
Thorazine, syrup	4.22	84	Sucrose
V-Cillin K, solution	3.00	60	Sucrose

Source: R. J. Feigel, "The Carcinogenic Potential of Liquid Medications," Special Care in Dentistry 2 (1982):20. Copyright © by The American Dental Association. Reprinted by permission.

Hidden sources such as medications add to the obvious sugar foods of which we are all aware: cookies, cake, pie, doughnuts, ice cream, Koolaid, candy bars, soft drinks, Jello-O, jam, syrup, and pudding. You can see how easy it can be to consume 75 percent to 80 percent of our sugar intake from processed foods and why our grandparents did no such thing, since few of the sugar-rich processed foods we now eat were available to them.

Comparing Different Kinds of Sugars

The "health food" industry has introduced a variety of supposedly natural and healthy sugars. But the truth is no sugar is very healthy. Sugar is basically sugar any way you take it.

Brown sugar is simply plain white table sugar (sucrose) with a bit of molasses added to it. Raw sugar is 99 percent sucrose. Corn syrup is the product of the incomplete hydrolysis of cornstarch. Corn syrup sweeteners consist mainly of dextrose (glucose), maltose, and more complex sugars. Add to these honey, molasses, maple syrup, malt syrup from cereal grains, date sugar, lactose (milk sugar), rice sugar, fig syrup, and fructose (a sugar found in fruits, berries, honey, and corn). True, fructose is a natural sugar, but it is also among the most highly refined and processed sugar products. All commercial fructose products are derived from corn, not fruit. All major soft drink producers are now using primarily high-fructose corn syrup in their formulas.[4] In fact, people with corn sensitivity or allergy find it quite difficult to avoid corn syrups, because these sweeteners appear in the majority of factory-prepared foods.

Most of our dietary sugars come from the sugars listed in table 17. The refined and processed sugars account for about 18 percent of our caloric intake. Six percent of our dietary calories come from the natural sugars found in milk (lactose), fruits (fructose), and vegetables such as starches, which eventually break down in our bodies into sugar. That's right, the average American's diet is 24 percent sugars.

Where That Sugar Hides

The tables in this section will give you some help in figuring out how much sugar is contained in the foods you buy at the store. Let's begin with cereals, in table 18. They range in percent of sugar calories from a high of 58 percent (Honey Smacks) to a low of 0 percent (Puffed Rice and Puffed Wheat).

Table 17

A Comparison of Various Sweeteners

	Relative sweetness	Calories/ tbsp.	Approx. cost/lb ($)	Nutritional quality*
White sugar	1	46	.35	Poor
Brown sugar	1	52	.75	Poor
Raw or tur- binado sugar	1	65	2.65	Poor
Fructose	2	56	3.00	Poor
Date sugar	0.6	75	5.00	Some B, Fe, Ca
Honey	1.3	64	2.50	Poor, but some K, Ca, P
Molasses	0.6	42	1.75	Good for Fe & Ca
Maple syrup	0.6	50	3.50	Good for Ca & Mg
Rice syrup	0.7	43	2.30	Good for K, some B, A, C, Ca
Barley malt syrup	0.6	N/A	2.35	Good for K, some B, A, C, Ca
Fig syrup	0.7	N/A	4.00	Poor
Corn syrup		57	.20	Poor

* B, A, C = vitamins B, A, C   K = potassium
  Ca = calcium   Fe = iron
  P = phosphorus   Mg = magnesium

Source: M. Barrett, "A Guide to Natural Sweeteners," Vegetarian Times (October 1985): 36. Reprinted with permission of Vegetarian Times, Oak Park, Illinois.

What these figures mean is that more than half of every tea-spoon of Apple Jacks and Honey Smacks consists of sugar cal-ories. You need to be aware of the sugar in even the "natural" granola cereals; in many, 20 percent to 25 percent of the calo-ries are sugar calories.

Our sugar consumption should not account for more than 10 percent of our total calorie intake.[5] Thus, any food in which sugar calories make up more than 10 percent of the total is by definition a less than healthy food. Of the eighty-five cereals listed in table 18, only twelve are less than 10 percent sugar calories. You can already see how the hidden sugar in our diets mounts up.

Many people, in attempting to eat a more healthy diet, have begun eating the flavored dairy products and yogurt. Unfor-tunately, these aren't always what they appear to be. The bad news is contained in table 19.

Now, just because the dairy products in table 18 contain too much sugar, it would not necessarily be wise to switch to other desserts. Table 20 lists the sugar content in a few other desserts.

Table 18

Refined Sweeteners (Sugar) Content
of Breakfast Cereals
(Serving size one oz.)

	Table sugar equivalent* (teaspoons)	Sugar calories as percent of total calories
GENERAL MILLS PRODUCTS		
Boo Berry	3.3	47
Count Chocula	3.3	47
Franken Berry	3.3	47
Chocolate Crazy Cow	3.0	44
Pac-Man	3.0	44
Strawberry Shortcake	3.0	44

Table 18 (continued)

Refined Sweeteners (Sugar) Content
of Breakfast Cereals
(Serving size one oz.)

	Table sugar equivalent* (teaspoons)	Sugar calories as percent of total calories
Trix	3.0	44
Cocoa Puffs	2.8	40
Lucky Charms	2.8	40
Cheerios, Honey Nut	2.5	36
Golden Grahams	2.5	36
Donutz, Chocolate flavor	2.5	33
Donutz, powdered	2.5	33
Buc Wheats	2.3	33
Nature Valley Granola, Fruit & Nut	2.0	25
Nature Valley Granola, Cinnamon & Raisin	1.8	22
Body Buddies, Brown Sugar & Honey	1.5	22
Body Buddies, Fruit Flavor	1.5	22
Kaboom	1.5	22
Nature Valley Granola, Toasted Oat	1.5	18
Nature Valley Granola, Coconut & Honey	1.5	16
Country Corn Flakes	1.5	11
Total	0.8	11
Total, Corn	0.8	11
Wheaties	0.8	11
Kix	0.5	7
Cheerios	0.3	4

Table 18 (continued)

Refined Sweeteners (Sugar) Content
of Breakfast Cereals
(Serving size one oz.)

	Table sugar equivalent* (teaspoons)	Sugar calories as percent of total calories
KELLOGG'S PRODUCTS		
Honey Smacks	4.0	58
Apple Jacks	3.5	51
Froot Loops	3.3	47
Cocoa Krispies	3.0	44
Sugar Corn Pops	3.0	44
Frosted Flakes, Sugar	2.8	40
Bran Buds	1.8	40
Frosted Krispies	2.5	36
Strawberry Krispies	2.5	36
Corn Flakes, Honey & Nut	2.2	33
Marshmallow Krispies	2.5	29
Raisins, Rice & Rye	2.5	29
All-Bran	1.3	29
Cracklin' Oat Bran	2.0	27
Frosted Mini-Wheats, Sugar-Frosted	1.8	25
Frosted Mini-Wheats, Apple-Flavored	1.8	25
Nutri-Grain, Wheat & Raisins	2.0	23
40% Bran Flakes	1.3	22
Crispix	0.8	11
Product 19	0.8	11
Rice Krispies	0.8	11
Special K	0.8	11
Corn Flakes	0.5	7
Nutri-Grain, Corn	0.5	7
Nutri-Grain, Wheat	0.5	7

Table 18 (continued)

Refined Sweeteners (Sugar) Content
of Breakfast Cereals
(Serving size one oz.)

	Table sugar equivalent * *(teaspoons)*	*Sugar calories as percent of total calories*
POST PRODUCTS		
Super Sugar Crisp	3.5	51
Honeycomb	2.8	40
Raisin Bran	2.3	40
Fruit 'n Fiber	1.8	31
Raisin Grape Nuts	1.5	24
40% Bran Flakes	1.3	22
Grape Nut Flakes	1.3	20
Grape Nuts	0.8	12
RALSTON PURINA PRODUCTS		
Cookie Crisp, Chocolate Chip flavor	3.3	47
Cookie Crisp, Vanilla Wafer	3.3	47
Donkey Kong Junior	3.3	47
Cookie Crisp, Oatmeal Flavor	3.0	40
Sugar Frosted Flakes	2.8	40
Raisin Bran	2.3	36
Bran Chex	1.3	18
Crispy Rice	0.8	11
Corn Chex	0.5	7
Corn Flakes	0.5	7
Rice Chex	0.5	7
Wheat Chex	0.5	7

Table 18 (continued)

Refined Sweeteners (Sugar) Content
of Breakfast Cereals
(Serving size one oz.)

	Table sugar equivalent* (teaspoons)	Sugar calories as percent of total calories
QUAKER OAT PRODUCTS		
Cap'n Crunch	3.0	44
King Vitaman	3.0	44
Quisp	3.0	44
Cap'n Crunch's Crunchberries	3.3	43
Cap'n Crunch's Peanut Butter	2.5	31
100% Natural, Raisins & Dates	2.3	28
100% Natural, Apples & Cinnamon	2.0	23
Life, Cinnamon	1.5	22
100% Natural	1.3	17
Life	1.3	18
Shredded Wheat	0.3	3
Puffed Rice	0	0
Puffed Wheat	0	0

* *Figures for cereals include naturally occurring sugar in raisins and other dried fruits.*

Source: "Sweet Surprises," Nutrition Action *(October 1984): 11. Copyright © 1986, Center for Science in the Public Interest.*

Table 19

Sugar Content of Various Dairy Products

	Serving size	Table sugar equivalent (teaspoons)	Sugar calories as percent of total calories
Frozen yogurt, whole milk	4 oz.	6.1	62
Lowfat yogurt, fruit	1 cup	7.5	52
Frozen yogurt, Dannon fruit	½ cup	3.3	50
Frozen yogurt, Dannon, vanilla	½ cup	2.8	50
Vanilla ice milk	½ cup	3.4	48
Vanilla ice cream	½ cup	3.2	37
Yogurt, flavored	1 cup	4.1	34
Chocolate milk, 2%	1 cup	2.7	24

Table 20

Sugar Content of Various Desserts

Popsicle	1	4.5	100
Canned pears, heavy syrup	½ cup	3.6	59
Canned pineapple, heavy syrup	½ cup	3	54
Chocolate pudding, homemade	½ cup	4.4	39
Hunt's snack pack pudding, Vanilla	1 can	4.4	37
Orange sherbet	½ cup	2.8	33

Source: "Sweet Surprises," Nutrition Action (October 1984): 11.
Copyright © 1986, Center for Science in the Public Interest.

The sugar content of regular soft drinks is easy to list. In all of them, between 95 and 100 percent of their total calories come from sugar! This includes tonic water and ginger ale. In many other packaged beverages, such as Kool-Aid, lemonades, cocoa mixes, Hi-C grape, and Gatorade, 80 to 100 percent of the calories are sugar calories. Hi-C for our kids and Gatorade for our athletes can accurately be called nutritional disasters!

Most chewing gums, Life Savers, and jelly beans are 95 percent to 100 percent sugar. Candy bars tend to have a sugar content of 10 to 40 percent and are usually quite high in fat as well.

Sugar, like fat and salt, has sneaked into the American diet in many ways, causing many of us to develop an insatiable craving for its taste. But our desires and cravings can be eliminated! People who decide to stop using alcohol, nicotine, or caffeine often find months or years later that they have minimal to no taste for those substances. By decreasing your sugar intake, you will gradually decrease your desire for a sweet taste. Read on to see how to cure *your* sweet tooth.

Notes

1. J. Bland, "Weight Management and Its Relationship to Hungry Appetite and Satiety," *Complementary Medicine* 2 (1987): 5.
2. "Sugar: How Bad, Really?" *Medical Self-Care* (January–February 1986): 36.
3. Ibid.
4. M. Barrett, "A Guide to Natural Sweeteners," *Vegetarian Times* (October 1985): 36.
5. U.S. Department of Health, Education, and Welfare, Public Health Service, *Healthy People: The Surgeon General's Report on Health Promotion and Disease Prevention* (Washington, D.C.: U.S. Department of Health, Education, and Welfare, 1979), publication no. 79-55071.

Chapter 8

Eating Less Sweet Food and Loving It

"I could never give up sweets," Annie told me. "Why would I ever deprive myself like that?" Annie's protests echoed those common among people with alcohol, nicotine, or other drug addictions. Initially she had learned to reward or console herself with sugary foods, and she was now addicted to them. She couldn't imagine life without them. Sugary foods had become a major component in her life, and she was being controlled by them.

Diminishing the Craving

Like the millions of people who have given up the supposed pleasures of alcohol, nicotine, and other drugs, Annie and the rest of us can learn to diminish our desire for sweet foods. As discussed in the preceding chapter, it is probably true that human beings have always enjoyed sweets. Historians say that Neanderthal people liked honey. The wealthy people thousands of years before Christ found sweet figs and dates to be special treats. The key, however, is to remember that sweets have *never* been consumed in the amounts in which we now eat them. As would be true with alcohol or cigarettes, none of us would have problems with these substances if we consumed modest amounts occasionally. But you will have to agree that an average sugar consumption of more than two pounds every week is not a moderate amount.

Despite the fact that we have cultivated a *preference* for sweets into a *passion*, we can and must change the upward spiraling course of our consumption. We are already beginning to make wonderful changes with babies' diets. Many more women are now breast-feeding than twenty years ago. This helps keep the infamous bottle of sugar water away from baby's teeth and taste buds. Another positive change is that sugar is no longer a major additive in most commercial baby foods. Yet another healthy sign is that many parents are beginning to make their own baby foods. This, of course, is only a good idea if the parents are eating a healthy, whole-foods diet.

More and more parents are rejecting treats for their preschool children that contain processed sugar. Instead, they are substituting such snacks as fruits, vegetables, nuts, and whole-grain crackers, pancakes, and pizzas. Perhaps even Halloween can be transformed, from a time of candy bars and confectioneries to one of balloons, crayons, games, and puzzles.

To help reduce our overemphasis on sugar, the schools need to begin revising textbooks. A University of California study showed that in 40 percent of textbook pictures of children eating, the foods being consumed are sweets.[1] It is interesting that for many American children, 40 percent of their calories come from sugars, the same percent found in the textbooks. The study analyzed 1,600 reading and workbooks used in kindergarten through third grade. Sugar-rich foods were the only food group appearing in every reading text. The sugar-rich foods constituted 19 to 100 percent of all food pictures and 17 to 70 percent of all food words.

The objective of changing textbooks would not be to eliminate all references to sweets from the books. Rather, the proportion of sugar-rich foods portrayed needs to be reduced to reflect the sugar recommendations set by the U.S. Department of Health and Human Services.[2] Then only 10 percent of the pictures and words would involve sweets, not the 40 percent that presently exists.

Television bombards our children with ads for sugary foods. Children get most of their sugar in sweetened beverages, cereals, bakery and dessert goods, ice creams, and candy. On any Saturday morning, you can view numerous television ads for most or all of these foods. And advertising works! Why do we allow our kids to be exposed to messages that are steering them toward foods that are not good for them? You will recall that earlier I presented some evidence showing that excess sugar consumption decreases the body's ability to fight infection. Similarly, some research indicates that sugary foods can increase a child's susceptibility to illness.

Change is occurring, if slowly. Some school hot lunch programs are using fewer syrup-packed fruits and are decreasing the amount of sugar in many of their recipes. We still have a long way to go, but we are heading in the right direction.

We need to allow our common sense to guide us more often. Do we really believe what the U.S. Food and Drug Administration has been telling us — that with the exception of tooth decay there is no evidence that sucrose is a health hazard? The majority of my patients do not believe that, and I don't think the majority of Americans believe it either. We need to believe what our instincts and our experience have been telling us: that excess sugar consumption is probably harming our health.

Just as we as a society long denied the existence of alcohol problems in the United States, so we are currently denying the existence of sugar problems. We all need to become more educated about what sugar can do to our health. We need to pressure food producers by not buying sugary foods. We need to demand more good sugar-related research in our state-supported medical institutions. And we must apply pressure for improved school lunch programs and quit using our kids to eat up the American food surplus of fats, sweets, and salt.

Making the Change

Try a simple experiment. Go for fourteen days with almost no sugar and see how you feel. This means fourteen days without the obvious sugar-containing foods such as pop, cookies, and candy as well as the foods containing hidden sugars such as yogurt and ketchup. It also means avoiding most of the fruit sugars and dairy sugars. No more than two fruit servings daily provides a minimal amount of sugar and will not negate the experiment.

I have worked with more than 500 people who have tried this two-week elimination diet, and the majority have been pleasantly surprised at how they felt by day twelve to fourteen. If 100 people try it, about twenty will feel significantly better than they have in years. They will have more energy, be less moody and irritable, weigh less, have less PMS, be headache-free, and have less craving for sweets. At the other end of the spectrum, about twenty people will notice no change or may even feel a bit worse. The other sixty will notice some improvement in how they feel, but the change will not be quite as significant as in those top 20 percent who are the most sugar-sensitive individuals.

I sincerely believe that most Americans are willing to avoid sugars for fourteen days if they realize they have up to an 80 percent chance of feeling somewhat or remarkably better. I know that many of my patients have been willing to do it with great success.

If, after you have done the trial, you aren't sure whether being off sugar has helped you, try a rechallenge test on day fifteen. The rechallenge consists of consuming large amounts of sugar for one day followed by careful observation of how you feel for twenty-four to forty-eight hours afterwards. If you feel the same as you did on day fourteen, the sugar was not affecting you in any immediately discernible way. If some of your symptoms get worse, then sugar was probably a cause.

Continuing to abstain from all sugar beyond the two-week trial period is difficult and not really necessary. I recommend that certain people increase their sugar intake slightly after the two-week elimination trial period. They may begin to have an occasional fruit juice or dairy product and even some ice cream, cake, or other sweet, though these should be once-a-week treats rather than once-a-day ones, as may have been these patients' former practice. Other people find that they are unable to eat any processed sugar products at all, because once started they are unable to stop. These people are severely addicted.

The following is a list of steps to take to help you through the first few months of a reduced-sugar or no-sugar diet:

1. Take frequent, small meals up to six times daily. This helps regulate blood sugar levels.
2. Eat healthy whole-food snacks at any time (for example, raw vegetables, whole-wheat breads or crackers, rice balls, cereals).
3. Increase B vitamins for the first two or three months.
4. Take large doses of one specific B vitamin—niacinamide (B_3)—for a short time. This tends to cut down sugar cravings. I have patients take 500 mg twice daily for one month. If any nausea occurs, I have them stop, because high-dose B_3 can occasionally cause liver problems.
5. Take extra chromium, which increases glucose tolerance. You can get this either in brewer's yeast or in pill form. The trivalent chromium, 100 micrograms three times daily before meals for one month, can be helpful.
6. Do aerobic exercise regularly for twenty to forty minutes four or fives times each week.
7. Join or form a support group of at least two other people who can meet with you once or twice a week during that first month or two. Support from friends is vital.

Remember, if you avoid sugar completely for just two weeks, you will have gone a long way toward losing your addiction to sugar. You will begin to have more taste for real food flavors rather than for the sugary taste that masks so many of our foods. And you will start to feel better physically and feel more positive about yourself. Your new diet will then be even easier to maintain.

Notes

1. M. Spletter, "A Move to Melt Sugary Images in School Texts,"
   Medical Tribune (27 February 1985): 15.
2. U.S. Department of Agriculture and U.S. Department of
   Health and Human Services, *Nutrition and Your Health,
   Dietary Guidelines for Americans* (Washington, D.C.: U.S.
   Government Printing Office, 1985), Home and Garden
   Bulletin No. 232.

Chapter 9

Artificial Sweeteners:
Is the Cure Worse Than the Disease?

I first saw Laurie, age 23, about one year ago. She was extremely frustrated because of hives that had been recurring over the preceding six to eight months. Her doctor had told her that they were probably caused by nerves, so she had begun psychotherapy but to no avail. Upon questioning, Laurie told me she was drinking about three cans of diet soda daily. I advised her to stop all diet substances for two weeks. When she returned she was completely free of hives for the first time in six months. She then tried half a glass of a diet soda and the hives returned. Laurie was sensitive to NutraSweet.

When 32-year-old Cliff came to me, he had already had colon and stomach x-rays plus a proctoscopic exam. His symptoms were gas, diarrhea, cramps, and bloating. He had been diagnosed as having irritable bowel syndrome and came to me to find out if there was anything else he could do. A dietary history on Cliff revealed that he ate two rolls of sugarless mints and a couple of dietetic wafers daily as weight reduction aides; he also chewed two packs of sugarless gum each day. On my advice, he avoided those substances totally for two weeks, and within six days he was symptom free. On day fifteen he tried some of the gum and again developed the abdominal complaints. Cliff was sensitive to sorbitol! Sorbitol is both a naturally occurring and synthetically produced sweetener.

These two examples make it clear that sugar substitutes can be as detrimental to health as is sugar itself. As you might suspect, there is considerable controversy over whether sugar substitutes are completely safe, usually safe, or unsafe. As with many issues in our lives, this is something about which people need to inform themselves and then make up their own minds. My guess is that for most people minimal amounts of sugar substitutes (such as NutraSweet) are safe, just as minimal amounts of sugar are. Some small percentage of citizens are more sensitive to the sugar substitutes, however, and will end up with some side effects. I believe that women who are planning to become or are pregnant should be extremely careful of sugar substitutes. Let's explore the issue further by taking a look at each of the sugar substitutes in turn.

Saccharin

Saccharin was first synthesized in 1879 and was the primary artificial sweetener for more than sixty years. Since the 1950s, there has been much controversy about saccharin. At that time, three different animal experiments showed an increased incidence of bladder cancer with saccharin use. More animal studies in 1972 and 1977 again showed bladder cancer. Canada banned saccharin in 1977 and the U.S. Food and Drug Administration proposed a ban in this country but was overruled by Congress, which decided that labeling saccharin-containing foods would be sufficient.

The major known side effect of saccharin has been not health problems but rather a bitter aftertaste. Some people report stomach upset with saccharin use, but that effect has not been well documented. Saccharin's biggest problem is that its safety has not been firmly established. There is still lingering concern that it may cause cancer. The other major concern is the risk posed to the fetus if a pregnant woman consumes it. The use of saccharin has decreased significantly since 1983, when aspartame (NutraSweet) was approved for use in beverages.

Aspartame (NutraSweet)

The sugar substitute aspartame, whose brand name is Nutra-Sweet, was discovered in 1965. It was approved by the Food and Drug Administration as a tabletop sweetener in 1981 and for use in beverages in 1983. Because it lacked the bitter aftertaste of saccharin, it quickly became the sweetener of choice in diet soft drinks. The consumption of diet soft drinks has been rising dramatically in America ever since 1983.

Aspartame itself is not found in nature but is synthesized from methyl alcohol and two amino acids that occur naturally in food—phenylalanine and aspartic acid. These two amino acids are found in meats, fish, milk, and grains. Detractors, however, point to a basic difference between eating the foods that contain these amino acids and eating aspartame. During digestion, they say, the amino acids are released gradually along with other nutrients. With aspartame ingestion, the body receives quick bursts of just these two amino acids.

Aspartame proponents say that the amount of amino acids released is too small to cause any reaction except in people with the genetic disease called phenylketonuria (PKU). People with PKU have an inability to metabolize phenylalanine. That is why the Food and Drug Administration requires that all packages of foods containing aspartame carry a warning to PKU sufferers.

The other component of aspartame, methyl alcohol, also deserves mention. In foods, such as cereals, this substance occurs in combination with ethyl alcohol, which is basically its antidote. In aspartame, however, methyl alcohol stands alone and is potentially toxic. In fact, Dr. Woodrow Monte, from Arizona State University, says that the classic symptoms of methyl alcohol poisoning (seizures, blackouts, headaches, depression, memory loss, blindness, nausea, and gastrointestinal disorders) are identical to complaints lodged by people who believe their ill health may be linked to use of NutraSweet.[1]

Numerous investigations and reports continue to conclude that consumption of aspartame by most people is safe and not associated with serious adverse health effects. The only exception to this conclusion is in those individuals who need to control their phenylalanine intake.[2] Despite the existence of excellent reports by very learned researchers, I tend to be a bit skeptical. My skepticism stems from my memory of the numerous chemicals that we were assured were safe and that turned out later to be unsafe. One of these was diethylstilbesterol (DES) for pregnant women threatened with miscarriage. After being freely prescribed for some years, DES was found to cause cancer in the offspring of some of the mothers who took it. A few other drugs that followed the same route are listed below:

- Oraflex, an arthritis drug that caused more than 100 deaths in a short time
- Bendectin, a drug for nausea in pregnancy that may have caused congenital abnormalities in the babies
- Thalidomide, a drug used for anxiety in pregnancy that caused hundreds of children to be born without arms or legs
- Tetracycline, an antibiotic that can cause a yellow staining of the teeth in children
- Chloramphenicol, an antibiotic that can cause aplastic anemia and death
- Even aspirin, which can cause bleeding ulcers, Reye's syndrome in kids, and tinnitus (ringing in the ears)

These examples illustrate why I wrote earlier that it is important for each individual to learn as much as possible about the sugar substitutes and then make up his or her own mind. Let's take a look at some of the reported side effects of aspartame.

In February 1984, the Food and Drug Administration asked the Centers for Disease Control to help evaluate aspartame complaints. Investigators interviewed 517 of 592 people who had reported problems with aspartame from 1983 (when it was approved) to April 1984, and 45 percent of the interviews were examined in depth. Here are the results of those interviews[3]:

- 67 percent of those questioned had neurologic or behavioral symptoms, including headaches, dizziness, and mood alterations.
- 24 percent reported gastrointestinal symptoms.
- 15 percent reported allergic or skin symptoms such as hives.
- 6 percent reported menstrual problems.
- 9 percent reported a variety of other symptoms.

These patients were not given avoidance and rechallenge testing, so there is no proof that their symptoms were actually caused by the aspartame. It certainly is of interest, though, that in less than one year of use, almost 600 people reported problems to the Centers for Disease Control that *they* thought were associated with NutraSweet. Most people with food-allergy symptoms are not diagnosed quickly, either by themselves or by a physician, so to have this number self-diagnose in the first year seems quite significant to me.

A number of other studies have confirmed that aspartame does cause side effects in certain people. A healthy 22-year-old woman who consumed three to four cans of diet soft drink daily developed deep nodules (lumps) on her legs. They completely disappeared when she stopped drinking the diet pop and reappeared when she rechallenged herself by drinking it again.[4] To be fair, it is important to understand that a few other studies show NutraSweet causes no more side effects than a placebo (inert substance). That is why the subject of aspartame safety is so controversial.

Can seizures possibly be related to NutraSweet intake? A medical researcher in Massachusetts found three people, ages 42, 27, and 36, who developed grand mal (tonic-clonic) seizures while drinking large amounts of liquids containing aspartame.[5]

None had a history of previous neurological disorders. A patient of mine who decided to quit drinking his six beers every night and switched to six diet soft drinks started having grand mal seizures two months later. It is possible that people thus affected would have developed grand mal seizures anyway, since seizures do, of course, occur in adults who do not consume diet drinks. However, I think the cases described are a bit unusual and would recommend that the dietary habits be investigated of all adults in the United States who begin to have grand mal seizures with no previous history of neurological disorders. Such a study would give us a good idea of whether or not this group of people has a higher-than-normal aspartame consumption.

Do you recall Laurie, described at the start of this chapter, who developed hives? A physician recently reported that he had asked 83 people with hives lasting at least six weeks to abstain from aspartame for two weeks. Follow-ups two weeks later revealed that in fifty of those people the hives had completely disappeared, usually within the first week of avoidance. Twenty-two patients avoided the diet sweetener afterward and remained hive free. Another twenty-two challenged themselves with aspartame-containing products and experienced hive reactions again.[6] These are very impressive statistics.

The examples cited make it clear that despite reassurances from a large number of investigators, many people in the United States believe that aspartame is causing them some problems. It makes sense, then, that if you have any of the problems listed below, you should consider a two-week elimination diet. If you discover nothing, all you will have sacrificed is diet foods for two weeks. If the diet eliminates some symptoms or discomforts, it may turn out to be the easiest and least expensive medical cure you will ever have come across.

Here are the symptoms and problems possibly related to aspartame:

- allergy
- depression
- dizziness
- fainting
- headaches
- itching
- memory loss
- menstrual pains
- mood swings
- nausea
- seizures
- skin nodules
- skin rashes
- swollen voice box (Laryngeal edema)

Cyclamate

The sugar substitute cyclamate was discovered in 1937 and accepted by the Food and Drug Administration in 1953. It was a popular sweetener in the 1950s and the 1960s but was banned in 1970. Currently it is not in use in the United States but is used in forty other countries, sometimes in combination with saccharine. Cyclamate was banned in the United States because large doses are linked with bladder cancer in laboratory animals. There is also evidence suggesting that cyclamate may be a cancer promoter if not an actual cause. And there is some question as to whether this substance may damage the chromosomes and cause shrinkage or atrophy of the testicles.[7]

I think there are two important reasons to discuss cyclamate. First, it is a sugar substitute that was considered safe for use by all of us in the 1950s and 1960s but is now banned. Is it not possible that this will also happen with aspartame and other agents?

Second, there is a moral issue associated with cyclamate that bothers me personally. An American government regulating agency has decided that cyclamate is not safe for consumption by people living in the United States. Yet we feel comfortable marketing it to the people in forty other countries. This seems to me an expression of unjustifiable arrogance plus a failure to recognize the fact that all people of the world are our brothers and sisters.

Fructose

Fructose is a simple sugar that occurs naturally in fruits, berries, honey, and corn. It is a natural sugar but, when produced commercially, is also among the most highly refined of the sugar products. All commercial fructose products are derived from corn. High-fructose corn syrup is cheaper to produce and buy than sucrose and has been widely substituted for crystalline sugar in a majority of soft drinks.

As you might guess, fructose can cause some health problems. Since it comes from corn, people with corn allergies who eat fructose can have any of the symptoms that corn itself causes them, such as skin problems or respiratory diseases. In some people, fructose can also cause intestinal problems — diarrhea, bloating, abdominal pain, and gas. These symptoms are often diagnosed as intestinal malabsorption, irritable colon syndrome, or spastic colitis when the problem is actually a corn allergy.[8]

Other Sweeteners

Do you remember Cliff (at the start of this chapter), who was sensitive to sorbitol? He had had severe intestinal problems over a long period that went away when he quit consuming his diet gum, mints, and wafers.

Sorbitol, xylitol, and mannitol are sugar alcohols that occur naturally in some fruits but are mostly produced synthetically. Numerous studies have linked sorbitol to chronic abdominal symptoms such as pain, cramps, gas, diarrhea, and bloating.[9]

Can you even begin to imagine the number of people in the United States who have these symptoms? Even if 0.1 percent of the people with intestinal problems had a sorbitol intolerance, thousands of people could be helped if they were made aware that sorbitol was causing their problem.

Carob

Although carob is not a sugar substitute, it is a chocolate substitute, so it seems appropriate to discuss it here. Before it is processed, carob powder is only 1 percent fat but up to 48 percent sugar. By comparison, cocoa powder is 23 percent fat and only about 5 percent sugar.

Unfortunately, when the carob powder is processed it is mixed with saturated fats and additional sugar. In fact, some carob bars contain more saturated fat than a Hershey bar, and others contain more sugar than a serving of ice cream.[10] For these reasons, I encourage people to avoid carob as well as chocolate.

I do not like bearing bad tidings to those who have tried to become healthier by giving up chocolate for carob. But a point made previously in this book is relevant here: immoderate use of *any* substance can cause problems. Conversely, even "problem" foods rarely cause symptoms if taken infrequently in minimal amounts. Rather, it is our abusive pattern of overuse and excess amounts that leads to problems. Remember, just as millions of people in America have learned to break addictions to alcohol and nicotine, all of us have the ability to eliminate our dependency on sweets or artificial sweeteners. Sometimes, just knowing you will feel a whole lot better without a food makes eliminating it easier.

You can probably understand now why I get so excited about the topic of food and its relationship to health and disease. For

many people, ending an aggravating, expensive, and at times
debilitating symptom or disease is possible simply by eliminating a food. Go ahead! Try it! If some symptom is bothering you,
look it up in the index and find out what food(s) *you* might try
eliminating.

Notes

1. W. Monte, "The Aspartame Controversy," *Vegetarian Times*
   (July 1986): 40.
2. Council on Scientific Affairs, "Aspartame Review of Safety
   Issues," *Journal of the American Medical Association* 254
   (1985): 400; and F. M. Sturtevant, "Use of Aspartame in Pregnancy," *International Journal of Fertility* 30 (1985): 85.
3. "CDC Survey on Aspartame," *American Medical News* (23
   November 1984): 39.
4. N. L. Novick, "Aspartame-Induced Granulomatous Pannicu-
   litis," *Annals of Internal Medicine* 102 (February 1985): 206.
5. R. J. Wurtman, "Aspartame Linked to Seizures," *Vegetarian
   Times* (February 1986): 10.
6. A. Kulczycki, "Aspartame Allergy Confirmed in Five
   Patients," *Family Practice News* (September 1985): 4.
7. J. E. Goyan, "Critics Say Cyclamate Not So Sweet," *Medical
   World News*, (22 July 1985): 34.
8. W. Hasler et al., "Malabsorption Symptoms May Be Linked
   to Fructose, Sorbitol in Diet," *Family Practice News* (1
   August 1987): 6.
9. N. K. Jain, "Low Sorbitol Tolerance Found Prevalent," *Medi-
   cal World News*, (13 August 1984): 7; M. J. R. Ravry, "Too
   Much Sweetener May Cause Diarrhea," *Journal of the
   American Medical Association* 244 (1980): 270; and J. S.
   Hyams, "Sorbitol Intolerance: An Unappreciated Cause of
   Functional Gastrointestinal Complaints," *Gastroenterology*
   84 (1983): 30.
10. B. Leibman, "Candy Is Candy Is Candy," *Nutrition Action*
   (April 1982): 14.

IV

Fats—
Stopping at Just Enough

Do you have any of these problems?

Acne
Allergies
Angina
Arthritis
Atherosclerosis
Bloating
Cancer of the breast
Cancer of the colon
Cancer of the prostate
Cancer of the uterus,
 ovaries, or testes
Chest pain
Constipation
Coronary artery disease
Diabetes
Dizziness
Fatigue
Gout
Hearing loss
Heart attack
Hypertension (high blood
 pressure)

Impotence
Indigestion
Intermittent claudication
 (leg pains)
Kidney stones
Menopause too late
Menstruation onset too
 early
Menstrual cramps
Nephritis (chronic kidney
 disease)
Obesity
Osteoporosis
Peripheral vascular disease
Premenstrual syndrome
 (PMS)
Senility
Skin rashes
Stroke
Transient ischemic attack
 (TIA)
Vertigo (loss of balance)

If you have any of these diseases or symptoms, read on
to find out how they might be related to the amount
of fat in your diet.

Chapter 10

Symptoms, Diseases, and Dietary Fat

From the list you've just read, you can see that excess dietary fats might be at the root of a great many health problems. There is controversy regarding many of these potential effects of a fatty diet. In fact, there is even controversy over what a fatty diet is and whether some fats (such as polyunsaturated ones found in fish) are good for us to eat.

The American Heart Association considers a diet risk free when 30 percent of the daily calories come from fat. I believe that figure should be 15 to 20 percent, and nutrition expert John McDougall, M.D., states that only 5 to 10 percent of total calories should be fat calories. At present, in the average American diet 40 to 45 percent of the calories come from fat, a range well above the recommended levels.

What are the sources of fat in our diet? It is difficult to find exact figures, but estimates are as follows:

- meat (including fish and fowl), 40 percent
- spreads, 30 percent
- dairy products, 15 percent
- baked goods, 8 percent
- eggs, 3 percent
- other, 4 percent

From this list it is clear that a diet based primarily on grains, legumes, vegetables, and fruits will be very low in fat.

Before we go much further into the subject, it's necessary to distinguish among the kinds of dietary fats. There are four general groups:

1. Saturated fats, found primarily in animal products such as red meats and dairy but also in coconut, chocolate, and certain oils derived from plants (margarine, palm oil, vegetable shortening)
2. Monounsaturated fats, found in olives and olive oil
3. Polyunsaturated fats, found in vegetables and fish
4. Hydrogenated fats and oils, made by adding hydrogen to vegetable oils

Although polyunsaturated fat intake often lowers blood pressure and serum cholesterol, I do not recommend eating it except in minimal amounts. Polyunsaturated fats tend to drive cholesterol from body tissues into the liver, gallbladder, and bowel. This excreted cholesterol can cause increased gallstones, cancer of the colon, and other types of cancer. Also, since vegetable oils are 100 percent fat, I recommend only minimal use of them even though they are a vegetable food. Other high-fat vegetable foods to be aware of are olives, coconuts, avocados, almonds, peanut butter, sunflower seeds, and tofu.

It is true that controversy persists over the potential health problems related to fat intake and the healthfulness of certain types of fats. Still, the evolutionary evidence remains convincing. Remember that our ancestors ate a low-fat, plant-based diet for thousands of years. My clinical experience tells me that our bodies are not equipped to process excessive fat calories of any kind. But in this, as in any controversial area, you must be the final judge. The first step, of course, is to learn as much as you can about the subject.

Angina

Florence was a 53-year-old woman who had raised four children, had helped her husband run the family farm, had done a good deal of nursing in the coronary care unit of the local hospital, and was now working for the government as a monitor of regional hospitals. She loved her new job, but it was somewhat stressful.

She came to my office complaining of chest pains over the past few months. She knew it was classic anginal-type pain, but she refused to believe that this could be happening to her. She was not a smoker, was only twenty pounds over her desired weight, and had no family history of heart disease. Unfortunately, she had some risk factors for atherosclerosis (hardening of the arteries). She rarely had time to exercise. Her blood pressure was mildly elevated at 150/95 (again, the ideal is 120–130/80–85). She had been a helper and giver for fifty-three years and held within her some resentment about that. She ate a typical high-fat southern Minnesota diet, consuming 45 percent of her 1,800 daily calories in fats. She did not know her cholesterol level. When I had it measured, it turned out to be 264 mg/dl. An ideal cholesterol level is less than 200 mg/dl; 200–250 is mildly bad, 250–300 is moderately bad, and above 300 is very bad indeed.

An exercise stress test was positive for heart disease. Coronary arteriography showed 90 percent blockage of one vessel, 50 percent of another, and minimal blockage of a third. Florence decided to make some life-style changes with respect to her way of handling stress and resentment, her diet, and how often she exercised. One year later, she was taking no nitroglycerine, her cholesterol level was 204, her blood pressure was 135/85, and she weighed nine pounds less than when she first came to me. She also had no angina and said she had not felt better since she was thirty years old!

Simply describing the process of hardening of the arteries goes a long way toward explaining why the condition is risky. High levels of fat and cholesterol form small wounds in the walls of coronary arteries. These sores attract platelets and white blood cells attempting to heal the sores. The fat and cholesterol accumulate at the site, scar tissue is formed, and a swelling called plaque develops. As more plaque is formed, the artery becomes hardened with it, and that is called atherosclerosis.

Hardening of the arteries is a huge problem for people in most highly industrialized countries. The richer (economically) countries of the world usually have richer (fat-wise) diets. When people have more money to buy packaged, canned, and fast foods, those are the foods they tend to buy and eat. Most of these foods contain significantly more fat than natural foods that have not been packaged, canned, processed, or made at fast-food establishments.

Atherosclerosis can start even in the first year of life and *often* does start by young adulthood. Autopsies on 22-year-olds killed during the Korean War frequently showed significant plaque formation in the coronary arteries.[1]

Do not despair, though. There is excellent evidence that, just as smoking cessation often stops the progression of lung disease, lowering our fat consumption will stop the progression of atherosclerosis. In fact, some epidemiological and animal studies show that atherosclerosis may be *reversible* with a low-fat diet.[2] Just think of it! Many of those friends and relatives you know who are having $30,000 bypass surgery or who are on numerous heart medications might do much better by adopting different life-style patterns, and especially new dietary habits.

Cancer

Joe had a routine proctoscopic exam, and two polyps were found in his lower colon. One of them was cancerous. Joe was 62 years old and wondered why he had colon cancer at such a young age. Virginia was only 49 years old when a breast lump was found to be malignant. Why are so many Americans getting cancer? The National Cancer Institute believes that the vast majority of cancers (69 percent) are at least partially caused by what we put into our mouths (see figure 3).

Figure 3

Sources of Cancer

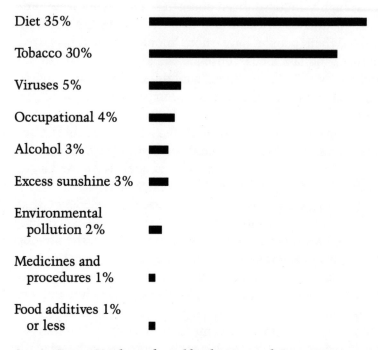

Diet 35%

Tobacco 30%

Viruses 5%

Occupational 4%

Alcohol 3%

Excess sunshine 3%

Environmental
  pollution 2%

Medicines and
  procedures 1%

Food additives 1%
  or less

*Source: From 1985 data released by the National Cancer Institute,
Washington, D.C.*

When I lecture on nutrition, I often ask audiences what percentage of cancer cases they believe relates to diet. More than 90 percent of nearly every audience guesses that fewer than 5 percent of cancers are diet-caused. The National Cancer Institute believes that diet, alcohol, and food additives may be responsible for 39 percent of our cancers, yet most Americans do not know that.[3] No one seems to know why such an important fact is not better known.

Even in 1986, almost every article on cancer prevention that I saw (whether in medical journals or in the popular journals for the public) failed to discuss primary prevention. They usually discussed only early detection (or what is now known as secondary prevention). Look at these typical examples:

Breast Cancer Prevention Recommendations

1. Self-exam each month
2. Physician exam each year
3. Mammography every one to five years, depending on age

Colon Cancer Prevention Recommendations

1. Yearly stool exam for blood
2. Yearly rectal exam by physician
3. Proctoscopic or sigmoidoscopic exam every one to five years, depending on age

As you can see, none of these tests will *prevent* even one case of cancer. The tests will only *detect* the cancer at an early stage. Since many of the cancers identified will have been growing for years already, early detection is frequently of no help.[4] This is surprising information, isn't it? True *prevention* of cancer would involve modification of an individual's life-style—with a large emphasis on diet.

Fats in our diet can truly cause a multitude of symptoms and diseases. Many of the problems are well proven to be at least partially the results of a high-fat diet. For others, the connection is more speculative but is considered a possibility. For example, medical science knows that fat causes hardening of the arteries but has not ascertained how fat relates to colon cancer. We do know that increased fat intake causes increased serum cholesterol levels in many people, and this increase leads to a build-up of plaque in various arteries throughout the body. When the plaque gets thick enough, it can actually block off the entire lumen (opening) of the artery so that no blood reaches the tissue the artery is meant to supply. That tissue then dies.

We call this tissue death a heart attack if it involves heart tissue and a stroke if it is brain tissue.

It's important to realize that when a heart attack occurs, it usually results from a condition that has been gradually evolving for many years. The plaque in the coronary artery has slowly been getting thicker. The actual attack itself occurs when the artery completely closes off and no more blood gets to the specific area of the heart served by the artery. An analogy from our daily lives might be a tub drain gradually becoming too plugged to drain the bath water. If we do not do something to clean out the debris in the pipes below the drain, we will one day end up with a complete blockage, with no water flowing through the pipes at all. Fat and cholesterol debris build up in our arteries in the same way. That's why I tell people who have angina or leg pains (called intermittent claudication) that they are really *lucky*. Their bodies are giving them a warning that they had better start changing their life-style habits or they will be having some serious problems in the near future. Most of us need a little "nudge" like that before we are willing to make significant life-style changes.

Another major problem caused by excess dietary fat is that it causes a build-up of estrogen in the body. Estrogen is a female hormone produced by the ovaries, adrenal glands, and certain other body tissues. It is extracted from the blood by the liver into the intestine. Fats encourage certain types of bacteria to grow in the intestine. These bacteria split up the estrogen molecules that are on their way toward elimination from the body, allowing the estrogen to be readily absorbed back into the body. Thus, excess fat leads to circulation of increased amounts of the powerful hormone estrogen throughout the body.

Below is a list of some of the diseases and symptoms that result at least partially from excess dietary fat causing plaque formation (i.e., hardening of the arteries), excess circulating estrogen, and other problems.

- *Angina pectoris.* This condition is caused by hardening of the coronary arteries (those that supply the heart).
- *Atherosclerosis.* Hardening of arteries anywhere in the body is called by this more generalized term.
- *Cancer of the breast.* Excess estrogen, which causes excess stimulation of breast tissue, can lead to this malignancy.
- *Cancer of the colon.* Many causes of this cancer are possible but one hypothesis is that excess bile is produced as the body tries to digest excess fats. These bile acids irritate the colon wall, which may eventually produce cancer.
- *Cancer of the prostate.* Excess estrogen production causes excess stimulation of the prostate and can lead to cancer.
- *Cancer of the uterus, ovaries, or testes.* These organs are also all responsive to estrogen and are abnormally stimulated by an excessive amount. This stimulation can lead to cancer.
- *Coronary artery disease.* As with angina, this is caused by hardening of the coronary arteries.
- *Diabetes mellitus (non-insulin-dependent-type diabetes).* High fat intake tends to cause increased body weight (fat contains nine calories per gram while carbohydrates and protein contain only four calories per gram). This type of diabetes is far more common in people who are overweight than in those who are of normal weight.
- *Dizziness.* Hardening of the arteries that supply the inner ear apparatus, which controls our balance, can cause this symptom.
- *Early onset of menstruation.* Excess estrogen can stimulate the ovaries and uterus to begin ovulation and bleeding earlier than is physiologically normal.

The normal age for beginning menstruation in societies with low-fat diets tends to be around age 16 or 17. In the United States and other places where high-fat diets are eaten, the normal age for menstruation to begin is about 12 or 13.

- *Hearing loss.* This also can sometimes be a result of hardening of the arteries that supply blood to the middle and inner ear apparatus.
- *Heart attack (myocardial infarction).* The cause of this serious and unfortunately common occurrence is similar to that of angina and coronary artery diseases: hardening and blockage of the coronary arteries.
- *Hypertension (high blood pressure).* One cause of this condition is generalized atherosclerosis, which decreases the size of the lumens in many of the body's arteries. When this condition is present, the heart has to pump harder to push the blood through the arteries adequately. The result is high blood pressure.
- *Impotence.* One cause of this problem is hardening of the arteries that supply the penis.
- *Leg aches (intermittent claudication).* This will often occur from hardening of the arteries that supply the legs.
- *Late menopause.* Excess estrogen can continue to stimulate the ovaries, causing ovulation to continue past the time that the ovaries are physiologically ready to stop.
- *Obesity.* This condition often results when a high-fat diet is eaten, since fatty foods have more calories per gram than protein or carbohydrate foods.
- *Peripheral vascular disease.* Like intermittent claudication, this usually is caused by hardening of the arteries to the legs.

- *Senility.* Hardening of the arteries to the brain can cause changes in mental abilities.
- *Stroke (cerebral vascular accident).* This is primarily caused by hardening of the arteries to the brain.
- *Transient ischemic attacks (TIAs).* These are short strokelike attacks that leave people wondering what happened. I compare TIAs to anginal chest pains that come and go and are caused by hardening of the arteries to the heart. TIAs are early warning signs that there are problems occurring in the arteries supplying the brain.
- *Vertigo (loss of balance).* One cause of this condition, which is similar to dizziness, is hardening of the arteries to the inner ear structures that regulate balance.

The preceding list is long and includes many serious problems. You may not believe it, but the list of fat-related problems does not end there. When people eat a high-fat diet, they are usually eating large amounts of meat and dairy products, which in turn usually means a high protein intake. Some diseases or symptoms can be linked to excess protein intake.

- *Chronic nephritis.* This can possibly be related to the kidneys working too hard to remove the excess protein from the body.
- *Gout.* This disease is a build-up of uric acid in a joint (often the great toe), which can cause excruciating pain and tenderness. It is thought to be caused sometimes when a large protein intake in the diet produces excess purines, the breakdown products of some proteins.
- *Kidney stones.* High meat intake can produce an excessive amount of oxalates, which make up many kidney stones. High protein consumption also increases calcium excretion, because calcium is

washed out with the large amount of protein. Since
a majority of kidney stones are made up of calcium
and oxalate, it is reasonable to believe that kidney
stones could result from increased protein intake.

- *Osteoporosis*. Thinning of the bones has many causes,
  one of which is excess urine excretion of calcium
  because of excess protein intake. I often tell my
  patients not worry so much about taking calcium
  pills and dairy products and to start worrying
  instead about how much calcium they're washing
  out of their body because of high protein consumption.

The preceding lists still do not exhaust the problems related
to high-fat and high-protein intake. Others are thought to be
at least *partially* due to high-fat consumption. I have seen dramatic improvements in many of these problems when patients
change their diet.

- *Acne*. Most dermatologists say that fat intake has
  nothing to do with this condition, but some believe
  that it increases sebum production, which leads to
  acne.
- *Allergies*. High on every list of foods potentially
  causing problems are some very fatty foods: milk
  and other dairy products, eggs, beef, and pork.
- *A bloated feeling after eating*. This often results
  from poor digestion of fatty foods.
- *Constipation*. Being "stopped up" can result from
  inadequate fiber intake, which in turn can result
  from a preponderance of meat and dairy products
  (which contain no fiber) in the diet.
- *Fatigue*. This may come from poor digestion of fatty
  foods in general, or it may come from an inadequate
  intake of vitamins and minerals owing to excess fat
  consumption and consequent inadequate consumption of nutrient-rich complex carbohydrates.

- *Gastrointestinal distress.* Gas, indigestion, or abdominal pains can result from either poor digestion of fats or allergies to some fatty foods.
- *Menstrual cramps.* These sometimes result from excess estrogen, which causes a hormonal imbalance in the body.
- *Premenstrual syndrome (PMS).* Again, excess estrogen produces a hormonal imbalance, which can produce PMS symptoms.
- *Skin rashes.* As stated before, some of the fatty foods are high on the list of possible food allergens. Generalized eczema (atopic dermatitis) in particular can be caused by intake of milk and other dairy products in sensitive individuals.

I will be the first to admit that the relationship of fatty foods to some of the problems in this last list is highly speculative. But most of the problems mentioned have been epidemiologically shown to be rare in populations eating low-fat diets. Also, in my twenty years of clinical practice, I have worked with patients with all these diseases and problems. Many of the conditions have been alleviated or resolved by diet modification such as increasing whole grains, beans, vegetables, and fruits. Improvement *can* be made! Our bodies have tremendous regenerative abilities. All they need is a chance to work.

Why Jack Sprat Was Healthy

Proving beyond a reasonable doubt that one diet is causing one disease is difficult. There are too many variables in studies trying to do this. Did the study subjects really eat exactly what they were supposed to? What else did they eat? Were they taking medications or drugs? Population (epidemiologic) studies are one way to help find diet-disease relationships.

Figure 4

Age-Specific Breast Cancer Mortality Rates in U.S. White Women and Japanese Women in 1980

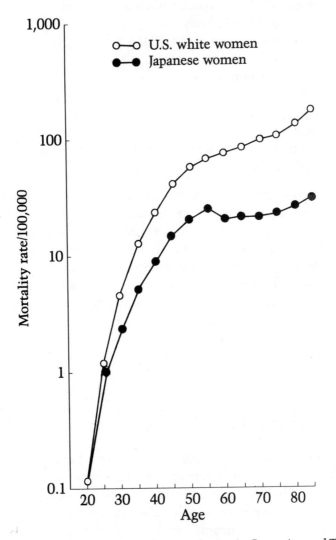

Source: E. Wynder, "Diet and Breast Cancer in Causation and Therapy," Cancer (October 1986): 1805.

Figure 5

Correlation Between Age-Specific Breast Cancer Mortality Rates (>55 Years) and Per Capita Fat Intake

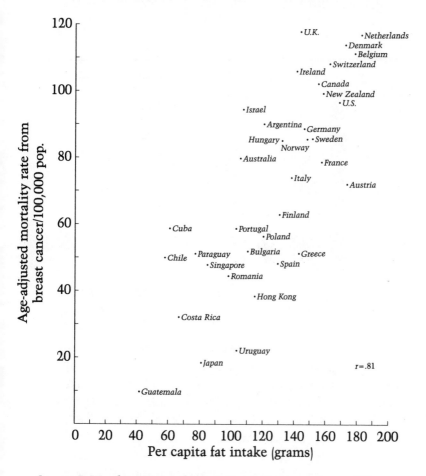

Source: E. Wynder, "Diet and Breast Cancer in Causation and Therapy," Cancer (October 1986): 1806.

Figure 6

Age-Adjusted Incidence Rates for Breast Cancer in
Caucasian, Japanese Issei (Japan Born), Japanese Nisei
(Hawaii Born) in Hawaii, and Japanese in Japan
(Osaka), 1973–1977

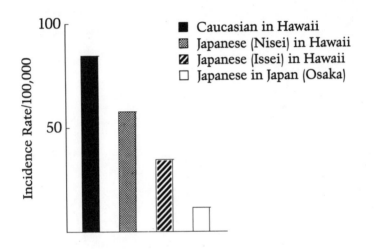

*Source: E. Wynder, "Diet and Breast Cancer in Causation and Ther-
apy,"* Cancer *(October 1986): 1807.*

The relationship between breast cancer and dietary fat intake
provides a good example of an excellent population study. The
women living in Japan have a very low rate of breast cancer compared with Caucasian women in the United States (see figure
4).[5] You can see that U.S. women have more than five times
more breast cancer after menopause than do Japanese women.
In fact, in almost every country, the incidence of breast cancer correlates with dietary fat intake — the more fat people consume, the higher is the rate of breast cancer (see figure 5).

Figure 5 shows that in countries with low fat intake (Gua-
temala, Japan, Uruguay), the breast cancer incidence is low.
Compare that to the high incidence in countries with high fat

intake such as the Netherlands, Denmark, Belgium, Canada, and the United States. It might occur to you that genetics, not fat intake, is the determining factor. That is a good thought but one that does not hold up to investigation. Look at figure 6 to see what happens to the rate of breast cancer in Japanese women when they move to the United States and begin to eat our high-fat diet. The incidence goes up remarkably.[6]

Breast cancer is not alone in its relationship to dietary fat consumption. Let's look at prostate cancer in U.S. and Japanese men (figure 7).[7] As you can see in figure 7, beyond age 70, the prostate cancer mortality is eight times greater in the United States than in Japan.

Why does increased dietary fat seem to promote cancer in the breast, prostate, uterus, ovary, and testicle? As mentioned earlier, dietary fat prevents adequate excretion of the body's excess estrogen. This estrogen is then absorbed back into the body, and the amount of estrogen in the bloodstream becomes excessive. Excess dietary fat also causes increased body fat, which will cause the body to produce *more* estrogen. Excess circulating estrogen overstimulates the growth and activity of hormone-responsive tissue, such as breast, prostate, uterus, ovary, and testicle tissue, and increases the risk of cancer.

Vegetarian women consume only about 30 percent of their calories in fats, while omnivorous (plant- *and* meat-eating) women eat about 40 percent of their calories as fat. The vegetarian women, therefore, usually have lower blood levels and higher stool levels of estrogen, meaning that these women are getting rid of more of their excess estrogen.[8] Vegetarians tend to have a lower incidence of all the fat-related cancers (breast, prostate, uterus, ovary, testicle, and colon).

The reason high dietary fat causes colon cancer is not clear. The disease may be related to the high fat intake itself or to high protein intake and/or low fiber intake, both of which are typical of a high-fat diet. Any one or all three of these factors may be a cause of colon cancer.

Figure 7

Age-Specific Prostatic Cancer Mortality Rate in U.S. White Men and Japanese Men in 1980

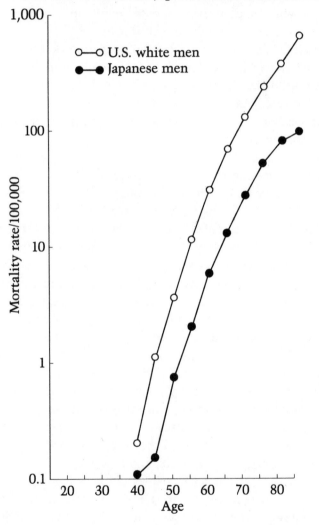

Source: E. Wynder, "Diet and Breast Cancer in Causation and Therapy," Cancer (October 1986):1805.

Hardening of the Arteries

All the atherosclerotic diseases (hardening of the arteries of the heart, brain, and legs) occur more commonly with a high fat intake. The lining of the wall of a blood vessel can be irritated and injured by high levels of fat in the blood. Muscle cells are then stimulated to overgrow the injured blood vessel lining as white blood cells and platelets race to the injured tissue to help repair it. Scar tissue then forms along with the

Table 21

Conditions Resulting from
Blockage of Various Blood Vessels

Blood Vessel Location	Symptom or Disease
Brain	Senility
Neck	TIA or stroke
Inner ear	Dizziness & vertigo
Middle ear	Deafness
Heart	Coronary artery disease with angina or heart attack
Penis	Impotence
Leg	Intermittent claudication or gangrene
Any vessels	Hypertension

Source: J. McDougall, McDougall's Medicine (Piscataway, N.J.: New Century Publishers, 1985), p. 101.

muscle cells, fats, and cholesterol. This swollen scar tissue is called plaque. The plaque gradually builds up, just as, in our earlier example, hair and debris accumulate in a shower drain. When the plaque builds up to a certain thickness, it begins to block the smooth flow of blood through that blood vessel. Depending on what blood vessel is being blocked, the result will be a symptom or disease, as table 21 shows.[9]

It makes little sense for society to spend $30,000 per person on coronary bypass surgery while spending almost nothing to help the public modify the typical American diet through education. Happily, people are now beginning to demand this type of education for this most serious problem!

Notes

1. W. F. Enos et al., "Coronary Disease Among United States Soldiers Killed in Action in Korea," *Journal of the American Medical Association* 152 (July 18, 1953): 1090–93.
2. R. Wissler, "Studies of Regression of Advanced Atherosclerosis in Experimental Animals and Man," *Annals of the New York Academy of Sciences* 275 (1976): 363; and M. Armstrong, "Regression of Coronary Atheromatosis in Rhesus Monkeys," *Circulation and Respiration* 27 (1970): 59.
3. The 1985 data are from the National Cancer Institute, Washington, D.C.
4. J. McDougall, *McDougall's Medicine* (Piscataway, N.J.: New Century Publishers, 1985), p. 30.
5. E. Wynder, "Diet and Breast Cancer in Causation and Therapy," *Cancer* (October 1986): 1804–13.
6. Wynder, "Diet and Breast Cancer."
7. Wynder, "Diet and Breast Cancer."
8. B. R. Goldin, "Estrogen Excretion Patterns and Plasma Levels in Vegetarian and Omnivorous Women," *New England Journal of Medicine* 307 (1982): 1542–47.
9. J. McDougall, *McDougall's Medicine*, p. 101.

Chapter 11

Eating Fewer Fats and Loving It

Dr. John Foreyt, a well-known expert on nutrition and obesity, recently gave a talk in Mankato, Minnesota, my home town.[1] He was asked about the value of the Pritikin diet (a high-fiber, low-protein diet with 10 percent fat calories). He said that he had been on that "extremely healthy" diet for a while and had felt great physically and lost some weight. He then went on to say that he had also been grouchy and irritable while on the diet and that he had really missed the fatty foods to which he had become accustomed.

That seemed to me quite a sensible and rational answer. But I balked when he said that because the diet was such a big change from his usual one, he (and probably most Americans) would not follow it over the long term, which led him to conclude that it was not a very useful diet. To me, that seemed like the Surgeon General of the United States saying that seatbelts really do save lives but since getting Americans to buckle up is difficult and inconvenient, let's just forget about the whole subject.

I use this example because it epitomizes the unwillingness of Americans to inconvenience themselves dietarily for better health. We *do* inconvenience ourselves in other ways to achieve better health—for example, by exercising and giving up nicotine and alcohol, but when it comes to changing our dietary habits, our resistance is strong. Many people want no special hardship imposed when it comes to eating. For example, hundreds of milk-drinking patients reacted quite vehemently when in the 1970s I began suggesting that they change to skim milk. They said they couldn't stand skim milk and that it would be impossible to switch. Gradually, the dietician and I persuaded them to try slowing cutting down the amount of fat in their milk. We urged them to mix whole milk and 2 percent for a while. Then they would drink 2 percent milk for a period. Next they would mix 2 percent and 1 percent milk, gradually change to 1 percent milk alone, begin mixing 1 percent and skim, and finally move on to consuming skim milk only. *Now* many of my patients tell me they cannot even drink 2 percent milk, much less whole milk. "It tastes like cream!" they say.

So, tastes *can* and *do* change, and dietary habits *can* and *do* change. Most people, if given the proper information, motivation, and support can gradually lower their dietary fat intake. Why not lower fat intake to a really healthy level (10 percent to 20 percent of total calories)? This change has a good chance of significantly improving how you feel and determining what diseases you get (or avoid getting).

Average fat intake in the United States is 40 percent to 45 percent of total calories. In 1979, the Surgeon General of the United States recommended that only 30 percent of one's total calories be from dietary fat.[2] This figure was reaffirmed in reports published in 1980 and revised in 1985.[3] Many people studying nutrition and its relationship to disease agree with Pritikin when he writes that if any disease or significant risk factors exists, only about 10 percent (and at most 15 percent) of one's intake should be fat calories.[4] If a person has few risk factors or diseases, then 20 percent fat calories may be all right.

Where Do Those Fats Come From?

Table 22 gives a general listing of approximate rankings of various foods as to the percent of fat calories they contain. You can see that the foods that are less than 20 percent fat—beans, whole grains, vegetables, fruits, and a few kinds of very lean meat and fish—largely make up the diet of our ancestors that

I keep touting. Note that the further down the list you move the greater are both the percentage of fat and the preponderance of meats, canned foods, and processed foods.

Tables 23 through 26 give a more detailed account of specific foods and their fat content. You can see that a diet composed primarily of grains, fruits, and vegetables is very low in fat. When dairy products (except for 1 percent and skim milk plus a few cheeses) are added, the fat content rises significantly. In choosing dairy products, it is important to remember that most cheeses are also high in salt, with between 150 and 400 mg of sodium per 1-ounce (2-tablespoon) serving.

As you scan table 24, showing the fat content of fish and meat, you will see why some people believe it is important to decrease the amount not only of red meat in our diet but all meat and some fish. These two items can easily account for the majority of fat calories.

If you're starting to wonder about that bologna sandwich or hot dog you had last week, your worst fears are justified. Seventy to 85 pecent of the calories in each of those products are fat calories. These foods are almost *total fat*. For a look at some of the processed meats, see table 25.

"I guess I won't make myself a bologna sandwich for lunch," you might say. "Maybe going out to eat will be better." As you can see in table 26, if you have any fast-food meat other than a Roy Roger's Roast Beef, you will probably be eating a meal with more than 50 percent of its calories in the form of fat. Remember: 30 percent fat calories should be our maximum intake.

To continue in another category, most frozen breakfast foods contain 35 to 72 percent fat calories. For instance, 35 percent of the calories in Nutri-Grain Waffles are fat calories; the same is true for Farm Blueberry Muffins. And many other frozen breakfast foods contain even more fat calories than these two products.

Table 22

Percent of Fat Calories in Foods

75% or more

Avocado
Bacon
Beef—choice grade of chuck
   rib, sirloin, and loin
   untrimmed, hamburger
   (regular)
Coconut
Cold cuts—bologna,
   Braunschweiger salami
Coleslaw
Cream—heavy, light, half-
   and-half, sour
Cream cheese

Frankfurters
Headcheese
Nuts—walnuts, peanuts,
   cashews, almonds, etc.
Olives
Peanut butter
Pork-sausage, spareribs,
   butt, loin, and ham
   untrimmed
Salt pork
Seeds—pumpkin, sesame,
   sunflower

50% to 75%

Beef—rump, corned
Cake—pound
Canadian bacon
Cheese—blue, cheddar,
   American Swiss, etc.
Chicken, roasted with skin
Chocolate candy
Cream soups
Eggs
Ice cream (rich)

Lake trout
Lamb chops, rib
Oysters, fried
Perch, fried
Pork—ham, loin, and
   shoulder (trimmed lean
   cuts)
Tuna with oil
Tuna salad
Veal

40% to 50%

Beef—T-bone (lean only),
   hamburger (lean)
Cake—devil's food with
   chocolate icing
Chicken (fried)
Ice cream (regular)
Mackerel

Milk, whole
Pumpkin pie
Rabbit, stewed
Salmon, canned
Sardines (drained)
Turkey pot pie
Yogurt (whole milk)

Table 22 (continued)

Percent of Fat Calories in Foods

30% to 40%

Beef — flank steak, chuck
pot roast (lean)
Cake — yellow, white
(without icing)
Chicken, roasted without
skin
Cottage cheese, creamed
Fish — flounder, haddock
(fried), halibut (broiled)
Granola

Ice milk
Milk, 2%
Pizza
Seafood — scallops, shrimp
(breaded and fried)
Soups — bean with pork
Tuna in oil (drained)
Turkey, roasted dark meat
Yogurt (low-fat)

20% to 30%

Beef — sirloin (lean only)
Corn muffin
Fish — cod (broiled)
Liver
Oysters, raw

Pancakes
Shake, thick
Soups — chicken noodle,
tomato, vegetable
Wheat germ

Less than 20%

Beans, peas, and lentils
Bread
Buttermilk
Cabbage, boiled
Cakes — angel food, sponge
Cereals, breakfast (except
granola)
Cottage cheese, uncreamed
Fish — ocean perch (broiled)
Frozen yogurt

Fruits
Grains
Milk, skim and 1%
Seafood — scallops & shrimp
(steamed or boiled)
Soups — split pea, bouillon,
consomme
Tuna in water
Turkey, roasted white meat
Vegetables

Source: Jane Brody, Jane Brody's Nutrition Book *(New York: Norton, 1981), pp. 76–77.*

Table 23

Fat Content of Fruits, Vegetables, Grains, and Dairy Products

	Serving size	% fat calories	Grams fat
MOST FRUITS	½ cup	0–8	0–0.5
VEGETABLES			
Most fresh vegetables	½ cup	0–6	0–0.5
Corn, canned	½ cup	13	1.0
Kidney beans	½ cup	15	0.5
Potato, fried in corn oil	10 strips	48	8.5
Avocado	½ medium	82	14.5
GRAINS			
Bread	1 slice	15	1.0
Bagel	1	5	1.0
Rice, brown or white	½ cup	0–4	0–0.4
Corn muffin	1	28	4
40% Bran Flakes	1 oz.	5	0.5
Quaker Granola	1 oz.	39	6
Shredded Wheat	1 oz.	8	1
Grape-nuts	1 oz.	0	0
Crispix	1 oz.	0	0
Quaker Oats, cooked	1 oz.	16	2
Pancakes, 6 in. diameter	1 cake	29	5.3
DAIRY PRODUCTS AND EGGS			
Milk, whole (3.3%)	1 cup	48	8
Milk, 2%	1 cup	31	5
Milk, 1%	1 cup	11	2.5
Milk, skim	1 cup	5	0.5

Table 23 (continued)

	Serving size	% fat calories	Grams fat
DAIRY PRODUCTS AND EGGS			
Milk, nonfat, dry (powdered)	1 cup	5	0.5
Half and Half	1 tbsp	90	2
Yogurt, whole	1 cup	48	7.5
Yogurt, low-fat	1 cup	14	3
Ice cream, 10% fat	½ cup	50–70	11
Ice milk	½ cup	15–27	2–5.5
Sherbet, 2% fat	½ cup	13	2
Egg, hard-cooked	1 large	62	5.5
Cheese, American	1 oz.	70–75	9
Cheese: blue, cheddar, Colby, Swiss, Monterey Jack, feta	1 oz.	70–75	9
Cheese, Velveeta	1 oz.	63	6
Cheese, cottage, regular	½ cup	29	5
Cheese, cottage, low-fat	½ cup	18	2
Cheese, cream	1 oz.	90	10
Cheese, Parmesan, grated	1 oz.	62	9
Cheese, mozzarella, part skim	1 oz.	56	5
Butter	½ oz.	100	11.5
Margarine	½ oz.	100	11.5
Margarine, diet	½ oz.	100	5.5
Oils, corn or olive	½ oz.	100	14

Source: Data collated from U.S.D.A. handbooks 8–10, 456, and 8–13, publications of the Dairy Nutrition Council (1986), and selected issues of Nutrition Action Healthletter.

Table 24

Fat Content of Meats

Food	Serving size	% fat calories	Grams fat
Poultry			
Light meat, w/o skin	3½ oz.	24	5
Light meat, w/ skin	3½ oz.	39	10
Dark meat, w/o skin	3½ oz.	34	8
Dark meat, w/ skin	3½ oz.	48	17
Fish (average of most fin & shell fish)	3½ oz.	25	4
Fish, canned in oil, drained	3½ oz.	37	8
Fish, canned in oil, undrained	3½ oz.	64	20
Fish, canned in water	3½ oz.	10	1
Veal (depending upon cut)	4 oz.	20–33	4
Pork loin, tenderloin	4 oz.	26	6
Pork (depending upon cut)	4 oz.	43–62	12–22
Lamb (depending upon cut)	4 oz.	30–53	7–16
Beef (depending upon cut)	4 oz.	26–82	6–48
Beef, ground, 80% lean	4 oz.	62	16
Beef, ground, 85% lean	4 oz.	58	14
Bacon	2 slices	90	6

Source: Data collated from U.S.D.A. handbooks 8–10, 456, and 8–13, publications of the Dairy Nutrition Council (1986), and selected issues of Nutrition Action Healthletter.

Table 25

Fat Content of Processed Meats

	% Fat calories	Fat (gm/2 oz.)	Sodium (mg/2 oz.)
5% FAT OR LESS BY WEIGHT			
Klement's Turkey Breast	18	1	522
Klement's jellied beef loaf	18	1	740
Eckrich Canadian Style bacon	26	1*	920*
Hormel barbecue flavored ham	36	1	N/A
Eckrich breast of chicken	23	2	840
Armour turkey ham	26	2	605
Eckrich gourmet loaf	26	2	780
Louis Rich roast turkey breast	26	2	460
Eckrich imported Danish ham	36	2	780
Oscar Mayer cooked ham	36	3	800
Oscar Mayer luxury loaf	32	3	667
6% TO 10% FAT BY WEIGHT			
Louis Rich turkey pastrami	51	4	540
Eckrich chopped ham	40	4	660
Hormel Canadian bacon	40	4*	630*
Klement's corned beef	43	4	740
Eckrich honey style loaf	45	4	700

Table 25 (continued)

	% Fat calories	Fat (gm/2 oz.)	Sodium (mg/2 oz.)
6% TO 10% FAT BY WEIGHT			
Oscar Mayer peppered loaf	45	4	812
Eckrich slender sliced beef	45	4	1,120
Eckrich slender sliced pastrami	45	4	720
Oscar Mayer ham roll sausage	46	4	670
Klement's honey loaf	46	4	740
Oscar Mayer New England sausage	46	4	732
Klement's yachwurst	47	4	740
Armour turkey meat loaf	45	5	313
Klement's barbeque loaf	55	6	740
11% TO 20% FAT BY WEIGHT			
Eckrich slender sliced smoked port	60	6	700
Eckrich slender sliced smoked chicken	60	6	780
Klement's chicken roll	56	7	290
Oscar Mayer cotto salami	72	8	608
Louis Rich turkey salami	60	8	500
Oscar Mayer pickle & pimiento loaf	59	8	777
Hormel little sizzlers pork sausage	79	9	172

Table 25 (continued)

	% Fat calories	Fat (gm/2 oz.)	Sodium (mg/2 oz.)
11% TO 20% FAT BY WEIGHT			
Louis Rich turkey bologna	75	10	450
Best's kosher beef franks	72	11*	370*
Best's kosher beef bologna	72	11	387
Hygrade chicken franks	76	11*	N/A**
21% OR MORE FAT BY WEIGHT			
Best's Kosher beef salami	74	12	387
Gwaltney chicken franks	78	13*	N/A
Hormel Prosciutto ham, boneless	70	14	1,004
Eckrich German brand bologna	79	14	700
Armour luncheon meat	80	16	600
Hillshire farm's smoked sausage	81	17	517
Oscar Mayer wieners	84	17*	581*
Oscar Mayer bologna	84	17	597
Oscar Mayer lean 'n tasty pork breakfast strips	71	20*	1,252*
Armour hard salami	75	20	1,050
Swift sizzlean pork	77	20*	760*
Swift pork brown 'n serve links	85	24	500

Table 25 (continued)

	% Fat calories	Fat (gm/2 oz.)	Sodium (mg/2 oz.)
21% OR MORE FAT BY WEIGHT			
Oscar Mayer bacon	80	30*	1,080*

* *Typical serving size is less than 2 oz.*
***N/A = not available*

Source: "What You Need to Know About Processed Meats," Nutrition Action Healthletter (May 1985): 11. Copyright © 1986, Center for Science in the Public Interest.

Table 26

Fat Content of Fast-Food Meat

	% fat by weight	% fat calories
Roy Rogers Roast Beef	1.7	13.7
Arby's Roast Beef	13.0	58.4
Hardee's Roast Beef	13.6	60.7
D'Lites D'Lite Burger	17.1	60.0
Burger King Whopper	20.1	66.6
McDonald's Quarter Pounder	20.2	66.5
Wendy's ¼ lb Hamburger	20.6	66.9
Roy Rogers Hamburger	21.3	66.0
Hardee's Hamburger	21.7	69.4
Denny's Dennyburger	22.3	70.0
Jack in the Box Jumbo Jack Hamburger	23.4	67.7
Carl's Jr. Famous Star Hamburger	23.6	70.0

Tests conducted by Lancaster Laboratories, Inc, Lancaster, PA. Moisture content of Roy Rogers Roast Beef was adjusted to account for gravy added to sandwich.

Source: "The Fat in Fast Foods," Nutrition Action Healthletter (June–July 1986): 6. Copyright © 1986, Center for Science in the Public Interest.

You can easily see that eating a diet limited to 15 to 20 percent fat calories would require one to focus on the whole, natural, unprocessed foods that humans have eaten predominantly for thousands of years. Our bodies have not adapted to the very different (high-fat) diet we now eat. A maladaptive physiologic process of disease in the form of cancer, heart attacks, hypertension, atherosclerosis, and possibly even osteoporosis and arthritis has been the result.

Many people have already significantly lowered their dietary fats and are finding that their long-term problems (such as angina and hypertension) are diminishing. Even on the short-term daily basis, my patients find that they have more energy and just feel better over all. My experience in dealing with large numbers of patients tells me that most are willing to suffer some inconvenience and irritability for a short period of time (while their bodies and taste buds adjust to a low-fat diet) in order to feel better each day. And the payoff is that they are significantly decreasing their risk of chronic degenerative diseases. The American diet *is* changing and will continue to change dramatically as people begin to understand its connection to their health and to demand lower dietary fat in foods.

Notes

1. J. P. Foreyt and K. Brownell, *Handbook of Eating Disorders: Physiology, Psychology, and Treatment of Obesity, Anorexia, and Bulimia* (New York: Basic Books, 1986).

2. U.S. Department of Health, Education, and Welfare Public Health Service, *Healthy People: The Surgeon General's Report on Health Promotion and Disease Prevention* (Washington, D.C.: U.S. Department of Health, Education, and Welfare, 1979), publication no. 79-55071, pp. 128–31.

3. U.S. Department of Agriculture and U.S. Department of Health and Human Services, *Nutrition and Your Health: Dietary Guidelines for Americans* (Washington, D.C.: U.S. Government Printing Office, 1985), Home and Garden Bulletin no. 232.

4. N. Pritikin, *The Pritikin Diet Pamphlet* (Santa Barbara, Calif.: Longevity Research Institute, 1978).

V

"Milk's Bad for Me?
You've Got to Be Kidding!"

Do you or your children have any of the symptoms or diseases listed below?

Abdominal pain (recurrent)
Acne
Allergies
Anemia
Angina pectoris
Anorexia or poor appetite
Asthma
Atherosclerosis
Bed-wetting (enuresis)
Behavior problems
Bloating
Blood in stools
Bronchitis (cough)
Canker sores
Colic
Colitis (irritable colon)
Constipation
Cramps
Crohn's disease
Dandruff
Dental cavities
Depression
Diarrhea
Ear infections (otitis media)
Eczema (atopic dermatitis)
Energy depletion
Excess phlegm and mucus
Fatigue

Flatus (rectal gas)
Gas in intestines
Headaches
Heartburn
Heart disease
High cholesterol
Hives
Hyperactivity
Indigestion
Insomnia
Irritability
Irritation of lips, mouth, or
  tongue
Joint aches
Multiple sclerosis
Muscle aches
Nausea
Pneumonia (recurrent)
Postnasal drip
Protein in urine
Restlessness
Sinusitis
Strep throat (recurrent)
Stuffy or runny nose
Tonsillitis (recurrent)
Ulcerative colitis
Ulcers
Vomiting

Any of these problems can be related to milk and dairy product consumption. Read further to find out why they occur.

Chapter 12

Milk—A Possible Culprit

Believe it or not, milk (often called "the perfect food") is the partial or total reason behind many people's vague complaints and even significant illnesses. You were probably astonished by the length of the list of symptoms and diseases that may be related to milk consumption. Well, so was I! Like most of you, I grew up with the belief that the more milk and dairy products we ate, the healthier we would be. In fact, this is still a commonly held belief among a majority of Americans. Strong, emotional, and significant debate continues between the majority of dieticians (who believe milk products are very important to good health) and those of us who believe that cow milk may be more harmful than healthful.

To help you in learning how specific problems you may be having could be related to milk, I have grouped the symptoms and diseases covered in this chapter into the following categories:

- gastrointestinal problems
- behavioral or central nervous system (CNS) problems
- skin problems
- respiratory problems
- heart problems
- other problems

All foods, including milk, are composed of carbohydrates, proteins, and fats. Thus, most problems associated with milk consumption result from the body's intolerance of one (or more) of the components of milk. That intolerance produces a symptom or disease in the body. Remember, cow milk is made for calves, not for humans.

Gastrointestinal Problems

Joan was a 42-year-old woman who had been diagnosed as having a nervous bowel. Other terms for this condition are *irritable colon, spastic colitis,* and *mucous colitis.* She was bothered with almost daily gas, bloating, loose stools, and abdominal cramps. Eight years after the diagnosis was made, Joan happened to read an article stating that milk sometimes causes these symptoms.

After stopping all dairy products for fourteen days, Joan found that she was entirely free of all her intestinal symptoms. On day fifteen, when she reintroduced dairy products (three glasses of milk and a bowl of ice cream), the gas, loose stools, bloating, and cramps returned worse than before.

Since Joan's father was a dairy farmer, she had trouble believing that the dairy products she had been raised on were the source of her problems, so she came to me for advice. I gave her articles to read about milk (lactose) intolerance. Twice more she tried eliminating dairy products in her diet. Each time, the gas and bloating would disappear, only to return when she reintroduced milk into her diet.

Joan called her regular physician to ask him why he had not mentioned milk intolerance as a possible cause of her bowel symptoms. He told her that milk problems are so rare she must be mistaken. He implied that she might be imagining things and that she had better not stop eating and drinking dairy products or she would end up with weak bones.

Is Joan's experience an isolated example? Not at all. Cow-milk consumption *does* cause gastrointestinal complaints in a large number of people. In fact, the majority of people in the world over the ages of 3 or 4 are lactose-intolerant.[1] Lactose, a carbohydrate, is the sugar contained in milk that gives it its sweet taste. Almost one-third of the calories in cow milk come from lactose.

Lactose has to be digested so it can be absorbed into the blood-

stream and be useful to the body (nutrients are useless if they
do not leave the intestines and enter the bloodstream). Lactose
digestion requires an enzyme called lactase. Let's look, in table
27, at just how common lactase deficiency is.

Cheese is one dairy product that is low in lactose (see table
28). Only 2 percent of cheese calories are from lactose, and
cheese causes few problems for lactose-intolerant people.
Unfortunately, most cheeses are quite high in fat and salt,
which means that eating them can cause other problems, as
we've already seen.

So, you say, cow milk can cause some bloating, gas, and
cramps. Those must be about the worst problems it causes,
right? Wrong. Let's look at the impressive list of gastrointestinal symptoms sometimes attributable to dairy consumption:

- abdominal pains,
  recurrent
- anemia
- anorexia or poor appetite
- bloating
- blood in stools
- canker sores
- colic
- colitis or irritable colon
- constipation
- cramps
- crohn's disease

- diarrhea
- flatus
- heartburn
- indigestion
- intestinal gas
- irritation of lips,
  mouth, or tongue
- nausea
- ulcerative colitis
- ulcers
- vomiting

Do you have any of these symptoms? If so, it will be easy to
determine whether milk is causing any or all of them. Just do
what Joan did. Eliminate all dairy products from your diet for
fourteen days. On day fifteen, reintroduce large amounts of
milk or ice cream. If you have lactose intolerance, you will feel
better without dairy products and worse when you reintroduce
them. This simple test may reveal the solution to a problem
that has bothered you for years.

Table 27

The Prevalence of Lactase Deficiency in Healthy Adults

Population group	% with deficiency
Filipinos	90
Japanese	85
Taiwanese	85
Thais	90
Indians	50
Peruvians	70
Greenland Eskimos	80
American blacks	70
Bantus	90
Greek Cypriots	85
Arabs	78
Israelis	58
Finns	18
Danes	2
Swiss	7
American whites	8

Source: F. A. Oski, Don't Drink Your Milk *(Syracuse, N.Y.: Mollica Press, 1983), p. 16. Reprinted with permission.*

Table 28

The Lactose Content of Dairy Products

	Amount	Lactose (gm)	% Lactose
Milk, whole	½ cup	6.0	30
Milk, 2%	½ cup	6.5	41
Milk, skim	½ cup	5.7	57
Yogurt, lowfat	½ cup	8.0	46
Cheese, cheddar	1 oz.	0.5	2

You may be thinking, "Wait a minute! I can go along with this gas and bloating, but are you saying milk can cause ulcers? My dad had ulcers and the only thing that *helped* him was milk." Well, milk *can* cause ulcers. Evidence in the past few years shows that in many people, milk actually keeps an ulcer from healing.[2] Your dad may have had years of ulcer problems *because* he kept drinking milk!

For people with lactose intolerance who want to continue to drink some milk, there is now a product called LactAid brand milk, made from 1 percent milk. A lactase enzyme is added to the milk so that lactase-deficient people have fewer gastrointestinal side effects. LactAid milk has a slightly sweeter taste than regular milk.

Allergy or sensitivity to milk *proteins* can also cause symptoms, just as lactose (carbohydrate) intolerance can. Among them are most of the same gastrointestinal problems just discussed. Discussion of other reactions to milk proteins follows.

Behavioral or Central Nervous System Problems

Brian was a 14-year-old boy who came to see me a few years ago. His mom was worried that Brian might have leukemia. Leukemia had been discovered in a cousin a few years earlier, and his symptoms were the same as Brian's. Over a period of two months, Brian had not slept well, was moody and irritable, often felt tired, had headaches, and had lost seven pounds. Brian and his mother revealed to me that he was under a lot of pressure from classmates to play football but that he was not really sure he wanted to. He had been out for football for about three weeks but was unable to go to practice most of the time.

Taking a careful dietary history, I learned that Brian drank about two quarts of milk every day, ate one or two bowls of ice cream four nights a week, and had cheese at least four times a week. After appropriate exams and blood tests, I suggested to Brian that he go two weeks without any dairy products. He pulled back in the chair, his pupils dilated, and he said that would be impossible. When asked why, he stated that dairy food was the only thing that made him feel good. I finally convinced Brian to try the two-week trial and saw him and his mother again in about twelve days. The first five or six days had been terrible for Brian, but after that he startèd feeling better. The last five nights he had slept all night and he had gained three pounds, had had no more headaches, was less fatigued, and was well on his way to recovery. Remember, this was a boy who had enjoyed dairy products for years. This story is a good example of how stress will often change the body's ability to handle a food that was previously handled with no problem. By the way, Brian decided to continue playing football.

James was a 10-year-old boy who saw me because of problems in school. The teacher had called James's parents to tell them that he was disruptive in class. The previous spring he had similar problems, but over the summer things seemed better. While I was taking his history, James was fidgety, had trouble concentrating on my questions, and argued with his mom numerous times. The history and exam also revealed that James wet the bed about three nights week and frequently complained of muscle aches. He loved milk and drank four glasses daily.

James agreed to avoid milk for two weeks. When I saw them three weeks later, both James and his mother were ecstatic about his improvements. James's teacher had even called his mother two days before, wondering what had happened to James because he was such a different child in class. He was no longer disruptive, he was paying attention, and he was doing good work. He had also stopped wetting his bed. Some of the proteins in milk apparently affected James's central nervous system, causing irritability, headaches, muscle aches, and bedwetting.

Dairy products are the leading cause of food allergies. Milk contains more than sixty different proteins, at least thirty-one of which may induce allergic reactions in humans.[3] Numerous studies report that one of the common areas of the body to be affected by milk allergy is the brain and central nervous system, which explains why such symptoms as irritability, fatigue, depression, and headache occur.[4]

The most difficult aspect of identifying an allergy that affects the central nervous system is that physical exams and blood tests rarely reveal anything to be wrong. So we physicians often assume that the problems must be psychological rather than within the nervous system itself.

Do you (or does your child) have any of the following problems, all of which *may* have been labeled psychological problems?

- bed-wetting
- behavior problems
- depression
- fatigue or lack of energy
- headaches
- hyperactivity
- insomnia
- irritability
- joint aches
- muscle aches
- restlessness

If so, I suggest you try to eliminate completely all dairy products for fourteen days and on day fifteen reintroduce lots of milk and milk products. You might be surprised to find that what you or your doctor called psychological, genetic, or stress-related problems were really caused by a milk-protein allergy or sensitivity. A fourteen-day dairy-elimination trail is a small price to pay to determine whether you are—or your child is—suffering from a milk-protein problem.

Skin Problems

Rachel was a 19-year-old Korean woman who had been adopted by an American family at age 5. She had had eczema since age 14. Despite the use of numerous cortisone creams, she was rarely without a rash on her legs. When I saw her for contraceptive advice, she mentioned the rash. It turned out that she drank 1 or 2 glasses of milk daily but had never liked it very well. Her parents had insisted she drink it, she said. When Rachel stopped all dairy products for two weeks, the rash started going away, and within two months she was completely rash-free for the first time in five years. When Rachel resumed eating dairy products again, the rash returned.

The skin is another area of the body that can be affected by milk-protein allergy and sensitivity. Rachel's case is a good example of this very frequent occurrence. Most physicians and numerous reports agree that milk is a frequent cause of eczema (called atopic dermatitis) and sometimes of hives.[5] Less evidence exists implicating milk as a cause of other skin problems such as acne and dandruff.[6]

Respiratory Problems

Toby and his parents had suffered through twelve of Toby's ear infections in the first two years of his life. The infections usually began with a stuffy or runny nose ("He always seems to have a cold!") and would end up as otitis media (infected middle ear). Antibiotic treatment seemed to be required constantly. When Toby stopped his dairy usage, the runny noses stopped and he only rarely had otitis media. The problem was that milk caused nasal congestion in Toby, which also caused blockage of his Eustachian tubes and subsequent middle ear infections.

The first thing I often tell any patient with a chronic stuffy or runny nose, excess phlegm, recurrent colds, sinus problems, or chronic cough is to try a 14-day dairy elimination diet. About one out of three people rid themselves completely of the long-standing problem this way. It's a simple and rewarding solution for both the patient and me.

Take a look at these common respiratory symptoms and diseases. Do you or your children have a problem with any them? If so, consider a milk allergy as a possible cause.

- asthma
- bronchitis
- ear infections (otitis media)
- nose stuffiness or runniness
- phlegm and mucus (excess)
- pneumonia (recurrent)
- postnasal drip
- sinusitis
- strep throat (recurrent)
- tonsillitis (recurrent)

Heart Problems

As we've seen, the milk carbohydrate called lactose and the many milk proteins can cause gastrointestinal problems. Also, the various milk proteins can cause brain, skin, and respiratory problems. The third component of milk is fat. You will recall from part IV that excess fat intake can contribute to plaque formation in arteries, causing hardening of those arteries. An interesting study involved ulcer patients, some treated with dairy products and some without. The ulcer patients who used dairy products experienced two to six times more heart attacks than those who used none.[7]

It would be wise to minimize your use of dairy products containing fats if you want to decrease your chances of having the following problems:

- angina pectoris
- atherosclerosis
- coronary artery disease
- heart attack (myocardial infarction)

Other Problems

Anemia means that the level of hemoglobin in the blood is too low. This condition is usually caused by blood loss. The use of cow milk in infants has been implicated in blood loss from the gastrointestinal tract and subsequent anemia.[8] This is the reason that mothers are strongly encouraged to breast-feed babies for the first year of life.

Nausea was mentioned previously with other gastrointestinal problems that can be caused or worsened by the use of dairy products. Nausea in pregnancy often responds particularly well to the elimination of dairy products. Maggie was 27 years old and in her fourth month of pregnancy. She had been having nausea with some vomiting since her second month. She was concerned because she was not able to eat much and had gained no weight during the pregnancy. Maggie saw a television program where a guest speaker mentioned that milk will often aggravate the nausea of pregnancy. She realized that before she became pregnant she usually drank only one glass of milk daily but that she had increased her intake to three glasses a day, thinking this was necessary. Maggie tried eliminating dairy products, and after seven days the nausea completely vanished and her appetite returned to normal. If she ate even small amounts of cheese or milk, the nausea returned. With appropriate dietary advice and calcium supplementation, Mary had a normal pregnancy and delivered a healthy baby.

Nephrosis is a chronic problem in which excess amounts of protein are lost in the urine because of a damaged kidney. One study showed that removing milk from the diet of some children with nephrosis caused them to stop losing protein.[9] When milk was added to their diet, the protein excretion increased markedly within one to three days. Further studies on this problem are scarce. I frequently wonder about the children I see for sports and school exams who are considered normal. About 10 to 20 percent of them spill (lose) protein on routine urine checks. There might be some interesting correlations in a study relating dairy intake and urine-protein spillage in presumably normal children.

Several other diseases are being investigated for their possible association with milk. There is no solid proof that milk is a cause of these — only anecdotal evidence. These conditions are multiple sclerosis, juvenile rheumatoid arthritis, amyotrophic lateral sclerosis (Lou Gehrig's disease), leukemia, and sudden infant death syndrome (SIDS). Much more research is necessary on all food products, not just dairy products, to determine whether links exists between them and significant health problems. But remember: milk can and does cause symptoms and diseases. It is not quite the perfect food most of us were taught it was. In the following chapter, we'll see why not.

Notes

1. F. A. Oski, *Don't Drink Your Milk* (Syracuse, N.Y.: Mollica Press, 1983).
2. N. Kumar et al., "Effect of Milk on Patients with Duodenal Ulcers," *British Medical Journal* 293 (1986): 666.
3. D. C. Heiner, "Issue of Prevalence of Cow's Milk Allergies Unlikely to Be Settled," *Skin and Allergy News* 12 (1981): 26.
4. A. Kahn et al., "Insomnia and Cow's Milk Allergy in Infants," *Pediatrics* 76 (1985): 880; J. Monro et al., "Food Allergy in Migraine," *Lancet* (July 1980): 1–4; M. B. Campbell, "Neurologic Manifestations of Allergic Disease," *Annals of Allergy* 31 (October 1973); 485–98; and H. Tryphonas and R. Trites, "Food Allergy in Children with Hyperactivity, Learning Disabilities and/or Minimal Brain Dysfunction," *Annals of Allergy* 42 (January 1979): 22–27.
5. A. J. Cant, "Food Allergy in Childhood," *Human Nutrition* (July 1985): 277–93; R. L. DeVillez, "Combined Therapy Said to Ease Eczema in Atopic with Food Sensitivities," *Skin and Allergy News* 15 (1984); F. Speer, "What to Do About Food Allergies," *Consultant* 12 (October 1973): 142–44; and M. Sampson and C. C. McCashill, "Food Hypersensitivity and Atopic Dermatitis," *Journal of Pediatrics* 107 (November 1985): 669–75.
6. J. McDougall, *The McDougall Plan* (Piscataway, N.J.: New Century Publishers, 1983), p. 50.
7. R. Briggs, "Myocardial Infarction in Patients Treated with Sippy and Other High-Milk Diets: An Autopsy Study of Fifteen Hospitals in the USA and Great Britain," *Circulation* 21 (1960): 538.
8. C. W. Woodruff and J. L. Clark, "The Role of Fresh Cow's Milk in Iron Deficiency," *American Journal of Diseases of Children* (1972): 124; and M. L. Halliday et al., "Cow's Milk and Anemia in Preterm Infants," *Archives of Diseases in Childhood* 60 (January 1985): 69–70.
9. J. M. Sandberg, "Food Allergy Cited as Cause of Relapse for Nephrotic Kids," *Medical World News* (2 April 1979): 18.

Chapter 13

Not Quite the Perfect Food

Milk certainly has some good things going for it. It is particularly rich in vitamin D, calcium, riboflavin, protein, and many other vitamins and minerals. Unfortunately, as the preceding chapter shows, milk can also cause a number of problems. Each of us needs to be aware of these potential problems so we can decide for ourselves whether to avoid milk and other dairy products completely or to use moderate amounts.

The dairy industry has done what is probably one of the best self-promotional jobs of all time. It has convinced an entire continent of people that milk is the perfect food and is necessary for good health. I believe that neither of these claims is true. Let's look at some of the reasons why people need to be more aware of what is wrong with the high consumption of dairy products.

Fat Content

Marvin had angina. Coronary arteriography showed that he had 90 percent blockage of one artery and 70 percent blockage of another. At age 37, he had coronary bypass surgery. When Marvin asked me why he was having these problems at such a young age, I explained to him that a possible cause was his fat consumption. Besides eating meat twice daily, he had been drinking one or two glasses of whole milk with every meal and having another at bedtime. He ate ice cream three or four times weekly, cheese about every other day, and occasionally yogurt. Marvin had been eating 3,300 calories daily, and almost 2,000 of them (60 percent of the total) were fat calories.

Let's review the figures for fat intake discussed in part IV. In the United States, fats account for an average of 40 percent to 50 percent of the total calories consumed. In 1979, the Surgeon General recommended that we decrease our fat intake to 30 percent of our total calories,[1] but the population has not achieved this goal. Many nutrition experts now suggest much lower fat consumption—for example, 20 percent of the total number of calories.[2] Nathan Pritikin, one of the most vocal advocates in the 1970s of the relationship between diet and disease, recommended that only 10 percent of our calories come from fats.[3]

The labeling on milk is tricky with respect to percentages. You need to learn to read it if you are to watch your fat intake. For example, you probably assume that in 2 percent milk, fat calories account for only 2 percent of the total calories. Unfortunately, that is not true (see table 29). Let me explain. One 8-ounce glass of 2 percent milk totals 240 gm and contains 145 calories. In the glass of 2 percent milk, there are 5 gm of fat. So 5 gm of fat out of a total 240 gm means the milk is, by weight, 2 percent fat (5 divided by 240). That is how the industry gets away with calling it 2 percent low-fat milk.

Table 29

The Fat Content of Milk

Type of milk	Fat content (% of total calories)
Whole	48
2%	31
1%	15
Skim	2–8

The tricky part is that fat has 9 calories/gm, so there are 45 total fat calories in the glass of milk (5 × 9 = 45). Recall now

that the total 8-ounce glass contains 145 calories. The 45 fat
calories account for 31 percent, not 2 percent, of the total.
Thus, almost one-third of the calories in a glass of 2 percent
milk are fat calories. Most people would not knowingly drink
one-third of a glass of fat with each meal. In summary:

$$8 \text{ oz. of } 2\% \text{ milk} = 145 \text{ calories} = 240 \text{ total gm} = 5 \text{ gm fat}$$
$$5 \div 240 = 2\% \text{ milk fat}$$
$$1 \text{ gm fat} = 9 \text{ calories, so } 5 \text{ gm} = 45 \text{ calories}$$
$$45 \text{ fat calories} \div 145 \text{ total calories} = 31\%$$

Drinking skim milk is good in terms of minimizing fat calories, but it increases the relative amount of milk proteins and
lactose you are consuming. As you will recall from the preceding chapter, milk proteins and lactose cause problems in some
people.

Various Chemicals and Other Substances in Milk

There can be other milk-related problems besides those
caused by the protein, carbohydrate, and fat in milk. Gary, age
38, had an irritating recurrent itch and rash over parts of his
body. His only known allergy was to penicillin, but he was
taking no medications. When Gary stopped eating all dairy
products, the itching and rash disappeared. We finally decided
that he had been getting small amounts of penicillin in his dairy
products, because when he drank locally produced penicillin-
free milk, he did not get the itching or rash.

Antiobiotics are commonly used to treat dairy cows for infections. It is possible for a person allergic to an antibiotic to
develop a milk sensitivity, manifested by problems such as
hives, itching, rash, sneezing, or asthma.[4] Such problems make
sense with hindsight, but their cause can be difficult to figure
out.

Another hazard associated with use of dairy products is their relatively high concentration of environmental toxins and contaminants. Since cows are large animals, dairy products are high on the food chain. This means that pesticides, industrial waste chemicals, and herbicides have more chance of accumulating in dairy products than they do in foods lower on the food chain (for example, grains and vegetables). This occurs because the cow eats large amounts of grains that are treated with these chemicals. People, on the other hand, eat much smaller amounts of grains, legumes, fruits, and vegetables, so their intake of pesticides and chemicals is much smaller than the cow's. Still, these toxins can cause immediate illness in people quite sensitive to them.[5] The possible long-term effects in humans are frightening. We are well aware that some chemicals, such as DDT, are cancer-causing agents.

Dairy products can also be contaminated with viruses that may cause leukemia. A leukemia-type virus is found in more than 20 percent of all dairy cows. In experiments on sheep and chimpanzees fed cow milk, some of the animals became infected and developed leukemia.[6] There is serious concern that these viruses may affect humans as well.

Another problem with milk is that the majority of dairy cows are pregnant while being milked (as soon as they give birth, they are bred again).[7] The cows, therefore, have increased levels of the hormone progesterone in their milk. We do not know if this extra progesterone affects humans or not, but our experience with problems caused by other hormones (such as diethystilbestrol, or DES, and estrogen) should be a warning. Also, progesterone breaks down in the body into testosterone, a male hormone, which can possibly have side effects such as acne.

A Lack of Fiber

The American diet is seriously deficient in fiber. One reason is that dairy products and meat have no fiber, and these foods compose a large portion of our daily fare. As I will discuss in part VI, low fiber intake is associated with a number of diseases, such as diverticulosis, colon cancer, and hemorrhoids.

Mineral Imbalance

One final problem with dairy products is that in some people they may be adding to a mineral imbalance in our bodies: excess phosphorus and insufficient calcium. Cow milk has a calcium-phosphorus ratio of 1.2 to 1 (while human breast milk has a ratio of 2 to 1). This means that when we eat and drink dairy products, we are taking in almost equal amounts of calcium and phosphorus. Evidence—albeit controversial evidence—suggests that phosphorus can combine with calcium in the intestinal tract and prevent the absorption of calcium.[8] Since popular foods such as meats, soft drinks, and baked goods all contain much more phosphorus than calcium, the concern about a mineral imbalance appears justified.

You are probably wondering by now what will happen to your bones if you don't drink "enough" milk. Let's explore that question in detail.

No Milk, Brittle Bones?

Recently, Ruth, a 57-year-old nurse, was admitted to our local hospital with a badly fractured ankle from a fall on our Minnesota ice. I visited her that evening to do a preoperative history and physical exam. She was scheduled for ankle surgery the next morning.

"Well, doctor, I guess I should have been drinking my milk all these years. The orthopedist says I have severe osteoporosis [thinning of the bones]." After doing a five-second relaxation exercise to control my Irish temper, I started discussing with Ruth what had really happened. The reason for my anger was that Ruth, like all of us, had been victimized by one of the most successful advertising ventures in history. The dairy industry has convinced all of us, including the American Medical Association and the American Dietetic Association, that milk is necessary for strong bones. So, here is Ruth—a very intelligent woman who has smoked one to two packs of cigarettes daily for almost forty years, who rarely exercises, who eats 45 to 50 percent fat calories and 20 percent animal-protein calories, who drinks six cups of coffee daily, and subjects herself to a lot of stress—still believing that her osteoporosis occurred because she did not drink milk!

Some studies do show that milk drinkers have less osteoporosis than those who do not drink milk. But rarely do these studies measure the quality of the subjects' diets, their exercise levels, and their other risk factors. There is reason to believe that if all causative factors were looked at, milk usage might be found to have very little impact.

Let's look at this possibility more closely. Most of the world's people do not drink milk, and they consequently take in less than half the calcium that we Americans are told we need. Yet these people, in general, have strong bones and teeth even into old age.[9] The highest rates of osteoporosis-related hip fractures in the world exists in the United States, Sweden, Israel, Finland, and the United Kingdom—countries that consume the *most* dairy products. In fact, a good way to measure the prevalence of osteoporosis in a country is to evaluate the incidence of hip fractures (see table 30).

The key to calcium's effect on the body is not how much calcium we put in our mouths but how much is absorbed by our bodies.[10] Adding more and more calcium to our diets or taking three or four calcium pills every day does not necessarily do much to increase the useful calcium in our body and bones, because the calcium has to be *absorbed* from the intestines.

There are several reasons why we Americans have trouble

absorbing calcium and tend to lose excess bone calcium:

1. High protein intake blocks calcium absorption.[11] With
   our high consumption of meats and dairy products,
   most Americans are eating more protein than they
   need, and calcium is not absorbed as well with a high-
   protein diet. The person eating a high-protein diet will
   excrete more calcium in the urine than a person eating
   a diet with less protein. Statistics show that the highest
   rate of osteoporosis-related hip fractures occurs in areas
   where protein consumption is highest (see table 31).
2. It has been thought for many years that the excess
   phosphorus in the American diet would bind calcium
   and prevent its absorption (see "Mineral Imbalance,"
   above). Some studies have disputed this theory and have
   shown that more phosphorus may actually *help* in calcium absorption.[12] Much more study must be done on
   the effect of the calcium-phosphorus balance.

Table 30

Incidence of Hip Fractures Compared with Intake of
Dairy Products in Several Populations

Country	Hip fractures per 100,000 population	Dairy intake (oz./person/day)
United States	98	16
Sweden	70	17
Israel	59	11
Finland	44	24
United Kingdom	43	15
Hong Kong	32	3
Singapore	20	4
South Africa (blacks)	6	0.4

Source: J. McDougall, McDougall's Medicine: A Challenging Second
Opinion (Piscataway, N.J.: New Century Publishers, 1985), p. 68.

Table 31

Incidence of Hip Fractures Compared with Protein Intake in Several Populations

	Hip fractures per 100,000 population	Protein intake (gm/day/person) Animal	Total
United States	98	72	106
Sweden	70	59	89
Israel	59	57	105
Finland	44	61	93
United Kingdom	43	54	90
Hong Kong	32	50	82
Singapore	20	39	82
South Africa (blacks)	6	11	55

Source: J. McDougall, McDougall's Medicine: A Challenging Second Opinion (Piscataway, N.J.: New Century Publishers, 1985), p. 68.

3. A lack of weight-bearing exercise causes increased loss of minerals from bones.[13] Until the recent fitness revolution in America began, modern people were significantly less active than their ancestors. This has been a major factor in bone demineralization and has led to the belief that we need more dietary calcium. In fact, we may simply need more exercise.

4. Cigarette smoking is a very strong risk factor for bone demineralization.[14] The exact mechanism by which this occurs is not yet known. It is known that smokers have a much higher incidence of osteoporosis than non-smokers.

5. A high-salt diet increases calcium loss in the urine.[15]

6. A high-sugar diet increases the spillage of copper into the urine, which has an adverse effect on bone mineralization.[16]

7. Alcohol and caffeine use, stress, inadequate sunlight, and use of certain medications, such as cortisone, antacids, thyroid pills, and diuretics, have all been implicated in increasing the rate of bone loss and adding to calcium depletion.[17]

It is evident from reviewing these factors that drinking more milk is not the answer to the complex problem of osteoporosis. Drinking milk or taking calcium supplements is an easy but inadequate substitute for the real and more difficult solution—life-style modification. Ruth's broken ankle was not simply a problem of inadequate milk intake. Ruth needed to make some major life-style changes, such as giving up smoking, exercising more, drinking less coffee, and learning to eat a low-fat, lower protein diet. Her usual calcium intake would probably then have been adequate.

How Much Calcium Is Enough?

The amount of calcium we take in may have little to do with how strong our bones are. The strength of our bones depends more on the many other life-style factors noted above.

The variation in calcium absorption is well illustrated by comparing infants fed breast milk with those fed cow milk. Breast milk contains 300 mg of calcium per quart, while cow milk contains 1,200 mg per quart. Yet the breast-fed infant absorbs more calcium than the infant fed cow milk. Clearly *more* calcium is not always better.

Another example of the adequacy of minimal calcium intake is provided by the African Bantu woman. She has no dairy intake but consumes 250 to 400 mg of calcium daily through the foods she eats. This is one-half the amount consumed by the average American woman. Yet osteoporosis is essentially unknown among the 10 percent of the female Bantu population that reaches more than 60 years of age.[18] Genetic protection has been considered as the reason but ruled out. When relatives of these same Bantu people migrate to more affluent societies and adopt rich diets, osteoporosis and diseases of the teeth become more common.[19]

Table 32
Calcium-Rich Foods

Item	Serving size	Calcium (mg)
Sardines with bones	3 oz.	372
Oysters	¾ cup	170
Salmon, canned with bones	3 oz.	167
Collard greens, cooked	½ cup	145
Tofu, processed	4 oz.	113
Spinach, cooked	½ cup	106
Shrimp, canned	3 oz.	100
Mustard greens, cooked	½ cup	97
Corn muffin	2 medium	90
Chili with beans	1 cup	90
Kale, cooked	½ cup	74
Baked beans	½ cup	70
Broccoli, cooked	½ cup	68
Orange	1 medium	55
Almonds	12–15	40
Egg	1 large	30
Green beans, cooked	½ cup	30
Whole wheat bread	1 slice	20
Peanut butter	2 tbsp	20
Lettuce	⅙ head	15
Spaghetti, cooked	1 cup	15
Orange juice	4 oz.	10
Apple	1 medium	10
Hamburger patty	3 oz.	10
Chicken	3 oz.	10
Rice, cooked	½ cup	10
Tuna	3 oz.	5

Source: N. Clark, "Calcium Content of Some Commonly Eaten Foods," Physician and Sports Medicine 12 (1984): 143. Permission to reprint is granted by Physician and Sports Medicine for nonprofit educational purposes.

Table 33

Calcium in Dairy Products

Item	Serving size	Calcium (mg)
Low-fat yogurt, plain fortified	1 cup	415
Part-skim ricotta cheese	½ cup	335
Low-fat milk (2%)	1 cup	300
Whole milk	1 cup	290
Buttermilk	1 cup	285
Vanilla soft-serve ice milk	½ cup	275
Swiss cheese	1 oz.	270
Cheddar cheese	1 oz.	210
American cheese	1 oz.	175
Vanilla soft-serve ice cream	½ cup	170
Vanilla ice cream	½ cup	100
Cream cheese	2 tbsp	20
Coffee cream	1 tbsp	15

Source: J. McDougall, The McDougall Plan (Piscataway, N.J.: New Century Publishers, 1983), p. 52.

The average American also consumes about 250 to 400 mg of calcium even without dairy products. This is because many nondairy foods also contain calcium (see table 32). If small amounts of dairy products are used, calcium intake jumps dramatically (see table 33).

The recommended calcium intake for Americans is now being debated (see table 34). Most government agencies are saying we need more calcium, but nutritionists such as John McDougall, M.D., and Jeffrey Bland, Ph.D., are saying we do *not* need to consume more calcium.[20] Rather, they suggest, we should lower our consumption of animal protein, phosphorus, salt, sugar, caffeine, alcohol, and nicotine, and increase our exercise. They believe these changes will enable us to achieve adequate calcium absorption without the use of dairy products or calcium supplements.

Sit down now and figure out your own calcium intake. If it averages about 800 mg daily, that is plenty unless you are pregnant or past menopause (if you are, you may need 1,200–1,500 mg). For others, even 400 mg daily is probably plenty if you eat minimal amounts of animal protein plus high-fiber foods, get plenty of exercise, and have healthful life-style habits.

You, your bones, and your health can do fine without milk. In fact, as you have discovered in this and the preceding chapter, you may even do better by avoiding most dairy products.

Table 34

Calcium Intake Recommended for the U.S. Population by Several Sources*

Source	Calcium (mg/day)
Research and experimental (minimum calcium need)	150–250
World Health Organization (adult minimum requirement)	400–500
Food and Nutrition Board (adult minimum requirement)	800
National Institutes of Health (recent proposal)	1,000–1,500

* Calcium intake in most populations of the world is 300–500 mg/day.

Notes

1. U.S. Department of Health, Education, and Welfare Public Health Service, *Healthy People: The Surgeon General's Report on Health Promotion and Disease Prevention* (Washington, D.C.: U.S. Department of Health, Education, and Welfare, 1979), publication no. 79-55071, pp. 128–31.
2. W. S. Creasey, *Diet and Cancer* (Philadelphia: Lea & Febiger, 1985), p. 206.
3. J. N. Leonard, J. L. Klofer, and N. Pritikin, *Live Longer Now* (New York: Grosset & Dunlop, 1974).
4. K. Wicher et al., "Allergic Reaction to Penicillin Present in Milk," *Journal of the American Medical Association* 208 (1969): 143; and M. Zimmerman, "Chronic Penicillin Urticaria from Dairy Products: Proved by Penicillinase Cures," *Archives of Dermatology* (January 1959): 1–6.
5. J. McDougall and M. McDougall, *The McDougall Plan* (Piscataway, N.J.: New Century Publishers, 1983), p. 36.
6. Ibid.
7. F. A. Oski, *Don't Drink Your Milk* (Syracuse, N.Y.: Mollica Press, 1983), p. 68.
8. Ibid.
9. Oski, p. 59.
10. B. E. L. Nordin et al., "The Relation Between Calcium Absorption, Serum Dehydroepiandrosterone, and Vertebral Mineral Density," *Journal of Clinical Endocrinology and Metabolism* 60 (April 1985): 651–57.
11. M. M. Linkswiler et al., "Calcium Retention of Young Adult Males as Affected by Level of Protein and of Calcium Intake," *Transactions of the New York Academy of Science* 36 (1974): 333; R. A. Chander et al., "Effect of Protein Intake on Calcium Balance of Young Men Given 500 mg Calcium Daily," *Journal of Nutrition* 104 (1974): 695–700; and R. M. Walker et al, "Calcium Retention in the Adult Human Male as Affected by Protein Intake," *Journal of Nutrition* 102 (1972): 1297–1302.
12. M. Hegsted et al., "Urinary Calcium and Calcium Balance in Young Men as Affected by Level of Protein and Phosphorus Intake," *Journal of Nutrition* 111 (1981): 553–62.

13. E. L. Smith, "Exercise for Prevention of Osteoporosis: A Review. *Physician and Sports Medicine* 10 (1982): 6; R. E. Laporte, "Can Increased Activity Cause Osteoporosis?" *Journal of Musculo-Skeletal Medicine* (February 1985): 51–56; and "Osteoporosis," *National Institutes of Health Consensus Development Conference Statement* 5 (1984).

14. H. W. Daniell, "Osteoporosis and Smoking," *Journal of the American Medical Association* 221 (1972): 509.

15. "Osteoporosis," National Institutes of Health.

16. J. Bland, "Calcium Pushers," *East West Journal* (January 1987): 70–73.

17. M. Notelovitz and J. Ware, *Stand Tall: The Informed Woman's Guide to Preventing Osteoporosis* (Gainesville, Fla.: Triad Publishing, 1982).

18. A. Walker, "The Influence of Numerous Pregnancies and Lactations on Bone Dimensions in South African Bantu and Caucasian Mothers," *Clinical Science* 42 (1972): 1891.

19. McDougall and McDougall, *The McDougall Plan*, p. 52.

20. J. Bland, "Calcium Pushers," *East West Journal* (January 1987); McDougall and McDougall, *The McDougall Plan*; and J. McDougall, *McDougall's Medicine*.

Chapter 14

Changing Your Milk-Drinking Habits

The most common questions I hear when I suggest trying a two-week dairy elimination diet are "What do I drink instead?" "What do I put on my cereal?" "Where will I get my calcium?" "You mean no cheese?"

Certain habits are comfortable for us and difficult to change. Dairy usage is one of these. Not only do we enjoy dairy products, but we have trouble finding good substitutes.

Is change possible? You bet it is! Many of my patients were drinking whole milk or 2 percent milk when I began discussing with them the disadvantages of dairy products. Most have gradually reduced their total milk intake and have changed the type of milk they use. As recently as 1980, if I even mentioned trying 1 percent or skim milk instead of whole milk, almost every patient thought it would be impossible, saying "That tastes like water!" Now, a few years later, the majority of my milk-drinking patients drink skim or 1 percent milk and believe that 2 percent or whole milk tastes terrible. "It tastes like cream!" "It's too thick!" is what I hear now. So, change *is* possible!

How much are you willing to change? Think for a moment of what our ancestors drank. There is reason to believe that until the last few centuries the majority of all liquid consumed by people was water. Nowadays, we believe we must drink juice, coffee, hot chocolate, sugared soda, diet soda, beer, wine, tea, distilled spirits, and milk. All of these liquids have a place in our lives, but they should be used occasionally, not daily. We generally accept that this is the case with alcohol, and we use it as an icebreaker at parties or a socially convenient way to share a special treat with friends. When alcohol usage becomes more consistent, however, as we are all aware, problems occur.

Each of the liquids I just mentioned is like alcohol, in that excessive use can cause health problems. The big problem is in defining what is excessive and what is moderate usage.

I was recently discussing soft drink consumption with the president of a local soft drink bottling company. He was upset about comments he had heard me make on a radio show regarding soft drinks. I said, "Fred, our problem is in our differing concept of moderation." He asked me what I meant. I said that soft drink moderation for him was drinking one or two cans of pop daily. He agreed. I said that my idea of moderation was one or two soft drinks weekly. Fred said, "That's terrible. That could mean twelve fewer cans of pop per person per week. My company would go broke!" And therein lies the reason that massive use of these various liquids is so highly promoted. (I can't think of anyone who would make money if we increased our water consumption—unless the bottled water craze continues to be popular.)

The best and simplest answer to the question, "What do I drink instead of milk?" is *water*. That is the only liquid we need for survival. In fact, we would survive much better if it were the only liquid we consumed.

For people eliminating cow milk who cannot get used to using water or juice on cereal, soy milk is a healthy alternative. It tastes a bit different from cow milk, but the difference is barely noticeable when soy milk is mixed with cereal. Soy milk is available at many stores both in ready-to-use and powdered form. You can also make it at home by processing soybeans. Soy milk is somewhat more expensive than cow milk but is very affordable when used in the small amounts needed for cereal. Since soy milk may seem too creamy if you are used to skim milk, try a half-and-half mixture of soy milk and water on your cereal at first.

For babies, breast milk is the ideal milk product for at least the first twelve months of life or until the mother or baby chooses to use a cup. For mothers who choose not to or are unable to breast-feed, I believe breast milk should be made available commercially. This system would be operational if people realized the importance of breast milk. Nursing mothers with excess milk could sell or donate their milk for babies who needed it. This has been done in France, where bottles of breast milk are delivered right to the homes of families who order it.

In the United States, premature babies are often fed breast milk in hospitals. (Newborn experts have long been aware that preemies do better on breast milk than on formula.) It seems strange that even though we know normal full-term babies experience less illness and less colic with breast milk than with formula, we make little effort to help those babies whose mothers are unable to or choose not to breast-feed. Somehow, our priorities seem a bit skewed on this subject. We will spend a quarter of a million dollars on a liver transplant to help one child, but we hesitate to spend a few hundred dollars to help the many nonbreast-fed babies have the healthiest possible infancy.

If breast milk is not available for a baby, then infant formulas such as Enfamil and Similac are better choices than cow milk. Formulas do not provide specific antibody protection against infection, but they do provide adequate nutrition for babies in the first year of life. The protein in formula more closely resembles that in breast milk than does the protein in cow milk, so there is less chance of allergy in babies fed formula than in babies fed cow milk.

For the child who is allergic to formula, several soy-based formulas are available (e.g., Isomil and Prosobee). If soy formula causes allergy, an elemental formula containing only amino acids can be used (e.g., Nutramigen, Pregestimil). These formulas can be purchased at pharmacies and are more expensive than regular formula.

Types of milk other than the normal dairy-case variety are basically milk products and have most of the same side effects.

Powdered milk can be whole or skim. It has simply had the water removed, and the skim variety has also had most of the fat removed, but the protein and lactose content remains the same. Sweetened condensed milk has had about half of its water content removed and sugar added to it. Kefir is a fermented milk that tastes like liquid yogurt. LactAid brand milk is treated with the enzyme lactase. As I wrote earlier, some people lack this enzyme, which helps digest the milk sugar lactose, in their digestive system. LactAid helps prevent such intestinal problems as gas, bloating, and loose stools resulting from lactose intolerance.

Yogurt is made by combining either skim or whole milk with a bacterial culture. The culture is then allowed to ferment, and the bacteria break down some of the lactose into its simple sugars, glucose and galactose—which our intestines may be unable to do. The culturing and incubation process may also modify the protein content and thereby reduce the chances of allergic symptoms. Of all the milk products, plain non-fat yogurt is probably the best for us. It is a low-fat food, the protein is less allergenic than in regular milk, and the lactose is partially broken down. Yogurt can also be made out of soy milk, which gives lactose-intolerant people another choice.

Nut-milk and seed-milk yogurts are made with rejuvelic, a fermented grain soaked in water. No cooking is involved, so these are good alternatives for people who avoid cooked foods. Goat milk can occasionally be tolerated by people who have problems with cow milk, probably owing to its slightly different amino acid composition. Goat milk is still too high in fat, protein, and lactose, however, for constant usage.

Raw milk is somewhat dangerous to use, because it may contain harmful bacteria or viruses. There are some reported cases of raw-milk drinkers having contracted *Salmonella* infection and becoming very sick. A few have even died.

A very healthy milk substitute can be made from rice or oats. The grain is cooked in water and then liquified in a blender or food processor. The result is a sweet liquid that works well on cereal.

Whey milk is beginning to be produced and may be a good alternative to other milks for some people. Cow milk is about 80 percent casein (curd) and 20 percent whey. Whey is what remains when casein is removed from skim milk. Human milk is just the opposite, with 80 percent whey. So whey milk more closely resembles human milk than does plain cow milk.

As you can see, a number of alternatives to cow milk are available, but only a few are really good. Most tend to cause at least some of the problems that regular cow milk does.

Remember, if you want to see whether milk is causing a health problem for you, stop *all* dairy products for fourteen days. If you notice a beneficial or positive difference, your body may be having problems with milk. On day fifteen, challenge your body with large amounts of dairy products and see if you notice any difference in how you feel. Table 35 lists foods allowed and not allowed on a strict, dairy-free diet.

Note: Hints for milk-free cooking include the following:
• *Use fruit juice, vegetable juice, or pureed fruits and vegetables in place of milk in cake, cookie, or quick bread recipes. Add one extra tablespoon of oil to the recipe.*
• *Use fruit juice or fruit sauces in place of milk on hot cereal.*
• *To make sour cream, mix ½ cup starch (corn, flour) with ¾ cup water, soybean milk, or goat's milk and stir in ¼ cup vinegar.*

Table 35
Planning a Milk-Free Diet

Foods allowed	*Foods not allowed*
Beverages	
Those made with water, fresh, frozen, or canned fruit juices, carbonated beverages	Those made with milk (skim, evaporated, condensed, buttermilk, dried, chocolate), all cream, Ovaltine, all instant chocolate mixes to which water is added

Table 35 (continued)

Foods allowed	Foods not allowed
Meat, fish, and poultry	
Beef, lamb, pork, veal, fish, poultry, baby food meats, bacon, ham	Prepared meats such as frankfurters, which may contain milk solids added as a filler, sausages, meat loaf, creamed chipped beef
Vegetables	
Fresh, frozen, canned varieties if served without butter, margarine, or cream sauce	Buttered or creamed vegetables
Potatoes and substitutes	
Potatoes, rice, macaroni, noodles, potato chips, French fries, spaghetti	Mashed potatoes if made with milk and butter, macaroni and cheese
Fruits	
Fresh, frozen, canned, or dried varieties if served without milk (can be sweetened)	Fruits with milk, cream, or whipped cream
Cereals and breads	
Any cereal to which no milk or milk products have been added during manufacture or preparation (fruit sauce or dried fruits can be added to cooked cereal), wheat, rice, oat, rye, corn, gluten, and soybean breads and rolls made at home without milk or milk products	Cooked cereals made with milk, Cream of Rice, commercial breads made with milk, doughnuts, popovers, pancakes, waffles, rusks, crackers

Table 35 (continued)

Foods allowed	Foods not allowed
Fats	
Olive or soybean oil, animal fat, olives, French dressing, mayonnaise, all whey-free dressings	Butter, margarine, salad dressing containing milk, cream, butter, margarine, or cheese
Soups	
Homemade without milk or milk products, broths, bisques, and chowders made with water	Any purchased (canned or dehydrated) or homemade varieties containing milk or milk products
Desserts	
Besides fruit, very few lend themselves to inclusion (for health reasons)	Cake or cookies made with milk, custards, ice cream, and pie crusts made with butter or margarine, pie, soft or cream-type puddings made with milk; sherbets; Bavarian creams, custards, chocolate candy or milk candies, caramels
Miscellaneous	
Spices, salt, pepper, plain herbs; chili powder, pickles, flavoring extracts, plain popcorn (no butter or margarine)	Gravy made with milk, cream, margarine, or butter, cream sauces, foods dipped in milk, butter, or margarine; biscuits, cakes, cookies, doughnuts, muffins, and pie crusts made from prepared mixes

VI

Processed Foods and Inadequate Fiber

Do you or your relatives have any of these problems?

Anal fissures
Appendicitis
Colon cancer
Constipation
Crohn's disease
Diabetes
Diverticulitis
Diverticulosis
Gallbladder disease
Heart disease
Hemorrhoids
Hiatal hernia
High cholesterol

High triglycerides
Hyperlipidemia
Hypertension
Inflammatory bowel disease
Obesity
Polyps, colon
Pulmonary emboli
Rectal cancer
Spastic or irritable colon
Thrombophlebitis
Ulcerative colitis
Varicose veins

If you know that one or more of these problems runs in your family, you will gain much helpful knowledge by reading the next three chapters.

Chapter 15

How to Mess Things Up Without Really Trying

You will recall that two diets were presented in the introduction to this book. Each contained the same basic foods from the four food groups. But the foods in Diet I were mainly processed foods that were less healthful than fresh foods for daily eating. They included a processed cereal, orange juice, canned corn, and potato chips. The foods in Diet II were primarily natural, unprocessed foods not changed much from their natural state. These foods were high in fiber and high in vitamins and minerals. They included a whole-grain cereal, an orange, corn on the cob, and a baked potato.

This chapter is all about what happens to our food when we process it. Does processing really make any difference in the food? Is whole-wheat bread really better for us than white bread? Bread advertisers discuss "enriched" white bread as if we were lucky to be able to eat such a fine product. A friend of mine compared white processed bread to a man who had been robbed of all of his clothes and money and then allowed by the robber to put on his pants so he could feel "enriched." Most of the fiber, vitamins, and minerals are stripped from the whole grain as it is processed into white bread (table 36). The maker of the white bread (the robber) then "enriches" the bread with some vitamins, including B vitamins, along with some iron and calcium (because these significant losses are compensated for, they are not listed on table 36). Unfortunately, at the end of the process the bread still lacks most of its original minerals and fibers.

When I talk to groups or patients about eating more whole grains, they almost always respond that they already eat dark

Table 36

Loss of Nutrients in Enriched White Bread as Compared with Whole Wheat Bread

Nutrient	% lost in white bread
Vitamin E	96
Vitamin B$_6$	82
Manganese	88
Fiber	78
Magnesium	78
Chromium	72
Zinc	62
Copper	58
Potassium	39

Source: "Termite's Delight, Eater's Digest," Nutrition Action Health-letter (September/October 1985): 9. Copyright © 1986, Center for Science in the Public Interest.

bread. Unfortunately, many dark or brown breads are not whole-grain breads. They are basically white breads with some molasses added to them. They usually contain more fiber than white bread but not as much as whole-wheat bread. I find that only about 10 percent of the brown breads available at the local supermarket are whole-grain breads. I also have trouble finding whole-grain noodles, macaroni, pizza crusts, pancake mix, and muffins. And, in our town, it is hard to buy more than a one-pound package of brown rice, while white rice is plentiful. All this means that we consumers are not asking for or buying very many whole-grain products.

What Is Fiber?

Processing depletes foods of important vitamins and minerals, and it also destroys much of the fiber. As table 36 shows, white bread contains only 22 percent as much fiber as whole-wheat bread. In the next chapter, you will learn why a lack of fiber in our diet is a major contributing factor to a multitude of medical problems and diseases. For now, let's just look at what fiber actually is.

Fiber is often referred to as *roughage* or *bulk*. It comes solely from plant foods and is that part of the plant not affected by our digestive enzymes. Fiber passes through our stomachs and small intestines virtually unchanged. When it reaches the large intestine (colon), part of it (called soluble fiber) is fermented by normal colon bacteria. This fermented fiber can then be partially absorbed and digested. The rest of the fiber (insoluble fiber) passes through the body with no fermentation, absorption, or digestion. The foods that contain the most soluble fiber are oat products, fruits, barley, and legumes (various types of beans and peas). The foods with the most insoluble fiber are wheat and rye products, vegetables, and most cereals.[1]

Meat, fish, and dairy products contain no fiber. Also, as table 36 suggests, processed foods, such as white bread, contain only minimal amounts of fiber. Given the typical American diet (see table 37), it is easy to see why we are a fiber-deficient country. We get 80 percent of our calories from fiber-poor foods, so we have to get most of our required fiber in just 20 percent of our food. However, we do not actually succeed in doing this. In the Western world, the average amount of fiber a person consumes in cereals and tubers (such as potatoes) fell from about 3.5 gm/day in 1860 to less than 2 gm/day by 1910 and to barely 1.5 gm/day by 1970.[2] Although fruit and vegetable fiber intake has increased, this does not compensate for the loss of fiber from cereals and tubers.

Numerous studies have documented the dietary changes that occur when primitive or rural people become urbanized and begin to have easy access to processed foods. In one study, when South African Bantus moved to an urban area, their fiber intake fell 80 percent, from 25 to 5 gm/day.[3] Also, as countries become

Table 37

Makeup of a Typical American Diet

Type of food (low fiber)	Percent of dietary calories/day
Fatty foods (primarily meats, fish, eggs, dairy, oils)	44
Processed grains (pastas, cereals, breads)	18
Processed sugars (soft drinks, confectioneries, other goodies)	<u>18</u>
Total of low-fiber foods	80

Type of food (high fiber)	Percent of dietary calories/day
Whole grains, fruits, vegetables, legumes	<u>20</u>
Total of high-fiber foods	20

Source: W. D. Manahan, "Dietary Analysis of 200 Patients at the Wellness Center of Minnesota," unpublished report, 1987.

more industrialized, the food consumed by the people of those countries becomes more processed. The dietary fiber intake of people in nonindustrialized countries is 60 to 140 gm/day, compared with the U.S. fiber consumption of 15 to 20 gm/day.[4]

Imagine holding a twenty-foot rubber hose from a second-story window of your house. Now, put feathers and bits of paper into the hose. You can well imagine that the hose will start to get clogged up and sluggish. In fact, we might even say the hose is constipated! Now take the same hose and put some sand and gravel into it. What happens? Suddenly, the sand and gravel race through the hose and emerge twenty feet below on the ground in almost the same quantity that entered it.

The hose in this instance is analogous to our intestines. When we eat primarily processed foods depleted of fiber (similar to the feathers), our food takes seventy to eighty hours to pass through us, producing small stool outputs of only 20 to 120 gm/day. Compare this to the very fast stool transit time (thirty hours) and large stool bulk (300 to 500 gm/day) of people in nonindustrialized countries, who eat a diet high in fiber (similar to sand and gravel in the hose).[5]

Vitamin-Mineral Depletion

As we've discussed, the processing of grains can deplete foods of vitamins and minerals. Unfortunately, canning and freezing can do the same to other foods. In fact, a can of corn, beans, or peas is frequently depleted of more than 50 percent of the minerals and more than 60 percent of some vitamins present in the food before processing (see table 38).

One interesting study allowed forty-six people to eat as much as they wanted from the four basic food groups for a single day. It was hypothesized that if given adequate exposure to the usually consumed foods from the four food groups, people would easily obtain adequate vitamins and minerals. But the

Table 38

Nutrient Loss in Processed Vegetables

	Vitamin B₆ (%)	Pantothenic acid (%)	Various minerals (%)
Canned vegetable	57–77	46–78	42–65
Frozen vegetable	37–56	37–57	35–50

Source: H. A. Schroeder, "Losses of Vitamins and Trace Minerals Resulting from the Processing and Preservation of Foods," American Journal of Clinical Nutrition, 24 (May 1971): 562–63.

findings actually showed that 67 percent of the forty-six participants did *not* obtain the recommended dietary allowance (RDA) for vitamins E and B_6 and for the minerals iron and zinc. And 34 percent did not obtain the RDA for folacin and magnesium.[6] This study highlights the difficulty Americans have with consuming adequate nutrients by eating even a balanced American diet. The available food choices are frequently low in nutrients and fiber.

The long-term effects of vitamin and mineral depletion in the diet have not been well studied. We are all aware that a significant depletion of certain vitamins causes diseases such as scurvy or beri-beri, but we need more studies similar to one done in 1980, which showed low thiamine (vitamin B_1) levels and early beri-beri symptoms in teenagers who ate the usual teen diets.[7]

In summary, eating mainly processed foods will lead to the following problems:

1. inadequate fiber intake
2. inadequate vitamin and mineral intake
3. increased incidence of various diseases.

It is this third item that will be addressed in the next chapter.

Notes

1. "Fiber at a Glance," *Environmental Nutrition* (October 1986): 6.
2. D. P. Burkitt, "Economic Development—Not All Bonus," *Nutrition Today* (January–February 1976): 6–13.
3. Ibid.
4. D. P. Burkitt, Speech given before Humanistic Health Society, University of Minnesota Medical Center, Minneapolis, 1982.
5. Burkitt speech.
6. "Nutritional Adequacy of the Four Food Groups," *Journal of Nutritional Education* 13 (1981): 46–69.
7. D. Lonsdale, "Thiamine Levels in Teenage Diets," *American Journal of Clinical Nutrition* 33 (1980): 205.

Chapter 16

Some Human-Made Diseases

Let us return to the analogy of the twenty-foot hose introduced in the preceding chapter. Which hose do you think will last longer and remain "healthier," the one with feathers in it or the one with sand and gravel poured through it? I would suspect that the hose blocked up with sludge from the feathers would probably start leaking and would wear out more rapidly. Similarly, when the gastrointestinal tract is blocked up, as may happen when a person eats a low-fiber diet, diseases occur more commonly than when the gastrointestinal tract is kept "free-flowing," as with a high-fiber diet.

Some gastrointestinal diseases occur frequently in North America but rarely in less-developed areas such as Africa.[1] A major difference between these two continents is the amount of fiber in the diet of their populations. Figure 8 compares the relative incidence in Africa and America of ten common diseases relating to the gastrointestinal tract or caused by gastrointestinal tract problems. As you can vividly see in figure 8, the ten very common American diseases are almost nonexistent among Africans. African whites tend to eat a different diet from that of most native blacks, one that is very similar to ours in America—high in processed foods and low in fiber. This results in a much higher incidence of gastrointestinal disease for the African whites.

People have suspected that blacks may have a genetic factor that protects them against the majority of gastrointestinal diseases. However, the argument about genetic differences becomes suspect when we examine the incidence of gastrointestinal diseases in American blacks. Look what happens! U.S. blacks who eat a low-fiber diet similar to that of U.S. whites

Figure 8

Relative Frequency of Various Gastrointestinal Diseases in Africa and North America

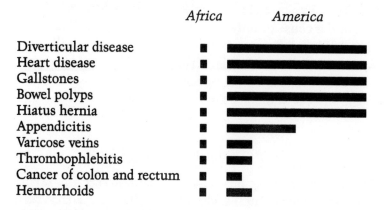

	Africa	America

Source: D. P. Burkitt, *"Economic Development—Not All Bonus,"* Nutrition Today *(January–February 1976): 7. By permission of Williams and Wilkens.*

now have the same incidence of these diseases as do the whites. Study findings such as these strongly support the belief that dietary habits have a tremendous influence on disease patterns. In summary, here is the evidence:

1. A large body of epidemiological findings (similar to those just presented) documents disease variations among different countries and races according to the amount of fiber consumed.
2. Empirical studies have shown marked variations in food transit time—for example, from three days in Westerners to about one day in rural Africans.
3. There are marked variations in stool size, from 20 to 120 gm/day in Americans eating a low-fiber diet to 300 to 500 gm/day in people eating a more natural, unprocessed diet.

The slow passage of stool through the intestine plus stools that lack bulk are believed to cause many medical diseases and problems. We will look at some of them in the following subsections. Be aware that some controversy still exists as to the role played by a lack of fiber in these diseases. Is it, say, 80 percent of the cause or only 10 percent of the cause? The exact effect of fiber deficiency is unknown, but very few will argue anymore that there is no relationship at all. You can learn about these controversies by reading the numerous papers and books on the subject of dietary fiber and disease.[2]

Constipation and Anal Fissures

Ed, a hard-working businessman, came to see me saying "Doc, I'm all blocked up. Besides that, I'm bleeding." Ed had been having about one stool each day until three months before his visit. At that time he had gone on a three-week business trip during which he rarely drank water, did not play his usual racquetball, ate no fruits or whole grains, and was under a lot of stress. Since that business trip, Ed had had to strain for a bowel movement every third or fourth day. Recently he had even developed occasional bleeding during a bowel movement.

You know what happened, don't you? Ed's stools had hardened owing to his decreased water intake, their bulk had decreased in size because of the lack of fiber in his diet, their speed of passage had decreased in response to the decrease in fiber and bulk, and his bowels had become sluggish from the lack of exercise. Stress can also affect many people's bowel-movement patterns; many people tend to suffer from loose stools with stress, but some, like Ed, experience the opposite effect. In Ed, the combination of factors resulted in severe constipation.

Ed's straining to pass the hard accumulated stool caused a tear at the anus (an anal fissure). Every time he had a bowel movement, the fissure, which had not quite healed, would tear again and bleed. Ed knew that rectal bleeding was one of the symptoms of colon or rectal cancer, so he became concerned. This worry motivated his visit to me in the first place. Diagnostic evaluation with rectal and proctoscopic exams, stool exams for blood, and a barium enema were all normal. Increased dietary fiber plus more water and exercise were all Ed needed to achieve normal bowel movements once again and to put his mind at rest.

Most physicians have significantly decreased their use of laxatives in nursing home patients by increasing the fiber in the residents' diets. Many also suggest to patients that they add oat or wheat bran to their diets, and they have seen good results. Constipation, truly a major American problem, is usually an easily remedied condition.

Hemorrhoids and Varicose Veins

Alice was upset with me. When I suggested to her that her diet might have something to do with her hemorrhoids and varicose veins, she told me emphatically that that was not the case at all. It was a family characteristic! Alice's mother had had both hemorrhoids and varicose veins, and now after the birth of Alice's second baby, she was having the same problems. It was clearly a genetic trait, said Alice.

I explained that there certainly is a genetic susceptibility to hemorrhoids and varicose veins but that, fortunately, some genetic susceptibilities can be altered by changes in life-style. You will remember, for example, that Japanese women rarely suffer from breast cancer until they adopt an American diet. And recall that vegetarians in America have less breast and colon cancer than their nonvegetarian neighbors. These people have altered their genetic susceptibilities (or nonsusceptibilities) to these cancers by changing their diet.

In the same manner, I told Alice, one can reduce hemorrhoid and varicose vein problems by making dietary changes. Recurrent straining for bowel movement causes increased pressure in the abdomen. Notice how tight your abdominal muscles get when you bear down. You can feel the pressure going down into your legs. This increased pressure will cause increased pressure in the veins in your anal area and legs. The veins gradually begin to dilate and swell, eventually resulting in hemorrhoids and varicose veins. If these problems continue, surgery is the only solution.

Two other significant diseases can relate to varicose veins and hemorrhoids. The first is deep venous thrombosis in the legs (called thrombophlebitis or blood clots). In this condition, a clot often forms as a result of poor valves and poor circulation in the varicose veins. The second disease is pulmonary emboli, which are blood clots in the lung stemming from the blood clots in the leg. These problems, like many we have discussed, are rare in developing countries. Clearly, some simple dietary preventive measures could save many Americans much pain and suffering.

Hiatal Hernia

A hiatal hernia, which is a tear or rupture in the diaphragm causing the stomach to protrude into the chest cavity, is a very common cause of heartburn, burping, acid indigestion, and pains in the chest and upper abdomen. The valve at the entrance to the stomach is supposed to allow food to drop into the stomach while preventing it from sneaking back up into the esophagus. If a hiatal hernia occurs, the upper end of the stomach protrudes into the thoracic cavity and the valve loses its ability to hold back the stomach contents. The stomach acids and digestive juices then infiltrate the very sensitive esophagus, causing a burning, soreness, or pain in the chest often mistaken for a heart attack.

On the basis of upper gastrointestinal x-rays, about 20 percent of Americans have been found to have hiatal hernias. (The incidence in India is 3 percent and in Africa 1 to 4 percent.[3]) The theory of D. P. Burkitt, a well-known researcher, is that the heavy straining from years of passing hard stools causes increased abdominal pressure, which in turn eventually causes the stomach to be pushed through the diaphragm and into the chest. Again, try pushing down for thirty seconds and notice how sore and tight you get in the upper abdomen just below your sternum.

All of this emphasis on fiber does not negate the fact that many other factors can also contribute to hemorrhoids, varicose veins, and hiatal hernia. These include, among other things, heavy lifting, obesity, pregnancy, genetics, and long hours of sitting or riding.

Diseases of the Colon and Rectum

Colon problems often attributed to inadequate dietary fiber include the following:

- anal fissures
- colon cancer
- diverticulitis
- diverticulosis (tics)
- inflammatory bowel disease (ulcerative colitis and Crohn's disease)
- polyps of the colon and rectum
- rectal cancer
- spastic or irritable colon

I will not discuss here most of the evidence implicating inadequate fiber as a casual factor in these diseases (see note 2 for some of the research involving these colon problems).

In general, current theories on why inadequate fiber intake contributes to gastrointestinal diseases cite as causative factors slow stool transit time, inadequate stool bulk, increased bile acid concentration, elevated levels of ammonia and long-chain fatty acids, altered gut bacteria, and abnormal pH values in the colon. Some of these factors may also relate to excess fat in the diet. When a person increases fiber intake, he or she almost invariably decreases fat intake. This is because the fatty foods (meats, dairy, oils) frequently lack or are low in fiber. Remember, fiber is that part of *plant*-based foods that humans cannot digest.

My guess is that everyone reading this book knows at least one person with one or more of the diseases or problems caused by lack of fiber. If you have a grandparent or parent over age 70, the chances of that person having diverticulosis is 20 to 50 percent.[4] Diverticulosis, although sometimes asymptomatic, is a major cause in older people of low abdominal pains, cramping, and bloating. Unfortunately, until very recently, we physicians encouraged people with diverticulosis to eat a low-fiber diet. This recommendation persisted for years, even after many articles were published suggesting that a high-fiber diet was better for diverticulosis.[5]

Even if we are not 100 percent sure that a high-fiber diet helps prevent most of the diseases listed, common sense directs us to eat in a manner more closely resembling that of our ancestors, who were rarely bothered by these problems. Their diet consisted primarily of vegetables, whole grains, legumes, and fruits. When meat was consumed, most evidence suggests that it was very low in fat, because it came not from deliberately fattened animals, as our meat does, but from animals that roamed long distances looking for food.

Just as inappropriate materials entering the lungs from outside the body (e.g., asbestos and cigarette smoke) cause lung disease (emphysema, bronchitis, lung cancer), so, it is highly suspected, can remnants of inappropriate food in the colon cause colon and rectal cancer, tics, polyps, colitis, fissures, and other colon diseases. Increased fiber in the diet dilutes harmful chemicals and shields the colon from their adverse effects. Also, as noted earlier, by increasing our fiber intake, we usually also decrease fat intake. In addition to the other positive effects of reducing fat intake, this step rapidly and dramatically reduces the amount of the carcinogens (cancer-causing substances) in the colon.[6] This effect is due to the fact that a high-fiber diet probably means a high consumption of vegetables, many of which cause the colon to produce enzymes that inactivate carcinogens.

It is fine to get periodic checkups by your doctor for colon and rectal cancer, ulcerative colitis, and other gastrointestinal diseases. But remember, those checkups, including x-rays, rectal exams, stool blood checks, and sigmoidoscopic exams, are for early detection, not prevention. True prevention will come only with life-style changes—one of the most important of which is renewed awareness of what we eat each day for the rest of our lives.[7]

Appendicitis

You may think after reading this subtitle that I have gone too far! Is he going to say that even America's number 1 emergency surgical procedure is related to our processed-food, fiber-deficient diet, you ask? Is it possible that some day we might not need to worry about appendicitis every time we or our kids have a stomachache? I certainly see a large number of children with the flu or some abdominal pain whose parents are worried that they might have appendicitis. Of course, given that they live in America, it just *might* be appendicitis!

There was evidence way back in 1920 that appendicitis was related to eating fiber-depleted foods.[8] Since the 1970s, extensive epidemiological evidence plus findings from a number of

fiber-intake studies have been collected.[9] It is postulated that
intake of fiber-low foods results in smaller, harder stools. Pieces
of the stool (called fecaliths) can obstruct the opening of the
appendix. This obstruction changes the pressure inside the
appendix and devitalizes its lining (the mucosa), which then
allows bacterial invasion and causes an inflamed appendix.

Diabetes and Obesity

There are two distinct types of diabetes. A small minority
of diabetics have type I (insulin-dependent) diabetes. This used
to be called juvenile diabetes, because it begins most frequently
in people under the age of 20. The onset of type I diabetes is
thought to have a minimal relationship to the person's weight
or diet. The vast majority of people with diabetes have type
II (non-insulin-dependent) diabetes. This type is closely associated with diet and obesity. It usually occurs sometime after
age 40, when people tend to put on excess weight.

In this section, I have combined diabetes and obesity because
it is impossible to discuss type II diabetes (the relevant type
here) without covering obesity. Since 1976 there have been
more than thirty reports documenting the beneficial effects
of a high-fiber diet in diabetic patients.[10] There remains very
little doubt that the low-carbohydrate diet recommended in
the past was basically incorrect. It had at least one positive
aspect, in that it encouraged diabetics to avoid some of the
sugars and processed foods (the simple carbohydrates). But
research has shown clearly that both diabetics and overweight
people need to increase their intake of *complex* carbohydrates
(starches) for better control of, and sometimes even *elimination of*, their diabetes and obesity.

Various theories have been suggested as to why a high-fiber
diet can help combat obesity:

1. The longer chewing required with high-fiber foods slows down the eating process and helps prevent over-eating.
2. Increased fiber intake slows the absorption of fats, so more calories leave the body in the stool.
3. Some types of fiber absorb water and retain sugar, thus slowing absorption of sugar calories by the body.

Remember, just because your grandmother, aunt, and mother had diabetes does not mean that you have to get it too. You may have a genetic susceptibility, but you also have information that may help you avoid ever getting it. That information is simple to sum up: You need to eat a diet high in fiber, low in fats, and low in processed foods. I know you can do it! Many Americans already are.

Gallbladder Disease

The role of fiber in gallstone formation remains speculative. Gallstones in westernized countries are mainly cholesterol-rich stones. When gallbladder bile becomes supersaturated with cholesterol, a stone forms. Factors favoring the cholesterol-rich bile are obesity and elevated serum levels of fat found circulating in the blood called glycerides. Gallstones are present in more than 10 percent of the adult population in America. In one Swedish study, 70 percent of women over 70 years of age had gallstones at autopsy.[11] In contrast, gallstones are almost nonexistent in rural areas of Africa.

So, even though the relationship between gallstones and fiber intake is unproven, there is much evidence accumulating to suggest that gallbladder disease is, at least partially, a result of a highly processed, low-fiber, high-fat diet.

Heart Disease, Hypertension,
and Hyperlipidemia

This nice alliterative title lumps together three of the major long-term disease problems in America. Most of us have a relative or close friend with at least one of these problems. Since the three major risk factors for heart disease are high blood pressure, high cholesterol, and use of nicotine, we could conceivably eliminate heart disease by changing what we put in our mouths (cigarettes or chewing tobacco, low-fiber processed foods, and fats).

Extensive studies have shown that diets rich in fiber can lower serum cholesterol concentrations by 20 to 30 percent.[12] This means that if your cholesterol level is too high (above 200 mg/dl), you can get it down to below 200 by increasing your fiber intake. Further, more recent studies have shown that the same high-fiber diet may lower elevated blood pressure.[13] Blood pressure is partially influenced by sodium, potassium, and calcium intake. A high-fiber diet generally includes less sodium and more potassium and calcium than the typical low-fiber diet. These alterations are all probably helpful for controlling and even preventing hypertension.

Remember that angina, heart disease, high blood pressure, and high cholesterol are not diseases that were dropped on us from "out there." We usually have *some* responsibility for their occurrence. Therefore, we have the power within us to do something about them. We have the power not only to prevent the continued worsening of high blood pressure, high cholesterol, and angina, but actually to reverse the course of these problems. A number of my patients have done so without medications or surgery:

- One man lowered his cholesterol level from 320 to 180 mg/dl.
- A woman decreased her triglyceride level from 1,200 to 120 mg/dl.

- A man maintained a blood pressure of 110/70 when it used to run a consistent 180/105.
- A man unable to walk more than half a block without anginal chest pain can now run a marathon.

It is these dramatic changes and others like them that have made my medical practice so exciting for me over the past ten years. Conveying my excitement to others has been my purpose in writing this book. I want everyone to know that he or she has the potential and ability to avoid or reduce the debilitating effects of a large number of symptoms and diseases that used to be thought incurable!

Notes

1. D. P. Burkitt, "Economic Development—Not All Bonus," *Nutrition Today* (January-February 1976): 7.
2. D. P. Burkitt and H. C. Trowell, *Refined Carbohydrate Foods and Disease* (New York: Academic Press, 1975); D. Kritchevsky, "Diet, Nutrition, and Cancer: The Role of Fiber," *Cancer* 58 (1986): 1830–36; J. W. Anderson and J. Jenkins, "Health Implications of Dietary Fiber," *American Journal of Gastroenterology* 81 (1986): 89; J. McDougall, *McDougall's Medicine: A Challenging Second Opinion* (Piscataway, N.J.: New Century Publishers, 1985); and D. P. Burkitt et al. "Dietary Fiber and Disease," *Journal of the American Medical Association* (1974): 1068–74.
3. Burkitt, "Economic Development."
4. J. R. Harrison, *Harrison's Principles of Medicine* (New York: McGraw-Hill, 1983).
5. A. Brodibb and D. Humphreys, "Diverticular Disease: Three Studies," *British Medical Journal* 1 (1976): 424–25; and J. Gear et al., "Symptomless Diverticular Disease and Intake of Dietary Fiber," *Lancet* 1 (1979): 511–14.
6. J. McDougall, *McDougall Newsletter* 1 (1987): 2.
7. P. Hill, *Cancer* 34 (1974): 815; and S. Ready, *Journal of Nutrition* 105 (1975): 878.
8. A. R. Short, "The Causation of Appendicitis," *British Journal of Surgery* 8 (1920): 86.

9. D. P. Burkitt, "The Etiology of Appendicitis," *British Journal of Surgery* 58 (1971): 658–99; A. Walker et al., "Appendicitis, Fiber Intake, and Bowel Behavior in Ethnic Groups in South Africa," *Postgraduate Medical Journal* 49 (1973): 187–93; and E. Arnbjornsson, "Acute Appendicitis and Dietary Fiber," *Archives of Surgery* 118 (1983): 868–70.

10. J. W. Anderson and C. A. Bryant, "Dietary Fiber: Diabetes and Obesity," *American Journal of Gastroenterology* 81 (1986): 898–906.

11. Burkitt, "Economic Development."

12. Anderson and Jenkins, "Health Implications," pp. 891–935; McDougall, *McDougall's Medicine,* pp. 203–225; and Burkitt, "Dietary Fiber," p. 1068.

13. J. Anderson, "Plant Fiber and Blood Pressure," *Annals of Internal Medicine* 98 (1983): 842–46; and O. Lindahl et al., "A Vegan Regimen with Reduced Medication in the Treatment of Hypertension," *British Journal of Nutrition* 52 (1984): 1120.

Chapter 17

Eating More Fiber—It's Easy!

My neighbor, Frank, found out the hard way that our intestines do not always adjust quickly to rapid dietary changes. We had a neighborhood picnic, and he overheard me telling someone else that one way to lose weight was to eat lots of high-fiber foods. He called my office and had the nurse send him a sheet showing the amount of fiber in various foods.

Frank is one of those people who gives 110 percent when he decides to do something. Consequently, in a few days time he had increased his daily dietary fiber intake 300 percent from 14 to 42 gm. Table 39 gives an example of the types of foods Frank used to eat and of those he began to eat on his new high-fiber diet.

Poor Frank quickly developed severe abdominal pains, distension, loose stools, and gas. The sudden increase in fiber was more bulk than his intestines could handle in such a short time. Frank called me a few nights later to ask what was going on with his body. He was upset because he was trying to become more healthy and lose weight and now he felt *worse* than he had in years.

Frank had not known that when increasing dietary fiber, it is a good idea to progress gradually. A monthly increase of 3 to 5 gm is probably fast enough. There is a huge variation in tolerance to fiber from individual to individual, so I instruct my patients to let their bodies be their guides. If increased fiber intake causes no symptoms, progression can be more rapid. If gas, pain, loose stools, or distension begin to occur, fiber intake should be decreased or stabilized. Remember that even healthy, positive dietary change is not without some risk.

What Is Fiber?

You will recall that dietary fiber comes only from plant foods. It is the part of the plant that goes through the stomach and small intestine unchanged. Digestive enzymes do not affect it. You will also remember that when the fiber reaches the large intestine (colon), the soluble fiber is fermented by bacteria living in the colon and can then be partially absorbed and digested. The rest of the fiber, insoluble fiber, passes through the body with no fermentation, absorption, or digestion.

Table 39

High-Fiber Meal Plan Versus Low-Fiber Meal Plan

High-fiber	Fiber (gm)	Calories	Low-fiber	Fiber (gm)	Calories
BREAKFAST					
Stewed prunes, 2 medium	3.9	40	Orange juice, ½ cup	0.0	40
All Bran cereal, ⅓ cup	9.0	70	White toast, 1 slice	0.8	70
Poached egg, 1	0.0	80	Margarine, 1 tsp.	0.0	35
Whole wheat toast, 1 slice	2.1	70	Poached egg, 1	0.0	80
Margarine, 1 tsp.	0.0	35	Skim milk, 1 cup	0.0	80
Skim milk, 1 cup	0.0	80	Water, 1 cup	0.0	0
Water, 1 cup	0.0	0			
TOTAL	15.0	375	TOTAL	0.8	305

Table 39 (continued)

	Fiber (gm)	Calories		Fiber (gm)	Calories
LUNCH					
Tuna salad			Tuna salad		
(½ cup tuna			(½ cup tuna		
+ 2 tsp.			+ 2 tsp.		
mayo)	0.0	190	mayo)	0.0	190
2 slices whole			2 slices white		
wheat bread	4.2	140	bread	1.6	140
Tomato slices,			Banana, 1 6"		
2; lettuce	1.0	10	medium	3.2	80
Carrots, 6			Yogurt, 1 cup,		
strips, raw	0.8	5	plain	0.0	150
Apple, 1			Water, 1 cup	0.0	0
medium					
with skin	3.3	80			
Water, 1 cup	0.0	0			
TOTAL	9.3	425	**TOTAL**	4.8	560
SNACK					
Popcorn,			Cupcake,		
3 cups (no			1 frosted		
butter)	1.2	75	(2½")	0.9	130
Apple juice,			Apple juice,		
1 cup	0.0	120	1 cup	0.0	120
TOTAL	1.2	195	**TOTAL**	0.9	250

Table 39 (continued)

	Fiber (gm)	Calories		Fiber (gm)	Calories
SUPPER					
Chicken, ½ breast (3 oz., no skin)	0.0	180	Chicken, ½ breast (3 oz., no skin)	0.0	180
Baked potato, medium with skin	3.0	130	Rice, white, ½ cup	0.8	70
Margarine, 1 tsp.	0.0	35	Asparagus, 4 medium spears	0.9	10
Spinach, ½ cup, steamed	5.7	25	Carrots, ½ cup steamed	2.3	25
Lettuce, 1 cup with ½ cup celery + 2 onion rings, green pepper	1.1	5	Coleslaw, ½ cup	1.7	60
French, low-cal dressing, 1 tbsp.	0.0	15	Dinner roll, 1 small	0.8	70
Bran muffin, 1 large	3.2	150	Margarine, 1 tsp.	0.0	35
Skim milk, 1 cup	0.0	80	Cantaloupe, ¼	1.6	40
Mixed fruit cup, 1 cup	3.2	80	Skim milk, 1 cup	0.0	80
Water, 1 cup	0.0	0	Water, 1 cup	0.0	0
TOTAL	16.2	700	**TOTAL**	8.1	570
GRAND TOTAL*	41.7	1,695		14.6	1,685

Both meals contain about 20 percent protein, 30 percent fat, and 50 percent carbohydrate.

Source: K. Cooper, "Compare Fiber Content," unpublished handout prepared by Aerobic Center, Dallas, TX, 1985.

The reason it is important to discuss these different kinds of fiber again is that some people have begun to take large fiber supplements in the form of such foods as wheat bran. They have probably read or heard that they need more fiber in their diets, so rather than moving toward naturally healthy high-fiber foods, they take supplemental wheat bran. This is an insoluble fiber that can interfere with mineral absorption. If a person were eating a diet of whole, unprocessed foods, the extra wheat bran would probably not be a problem. The normally healthful diet would most likely supply sufficient minerals to make up any deficit brought on by the extra fiber. What is more common, though, is for people to increase their wheat bran consumption but to continue eating their usual, highly processed American diet. A person doing this may be helping his or her constipation but depleting the body of important minerals.

The key to good health is balance. Some extra oat bran or wheat bran occasionally is fine, but the most helpful advice is to do what dieticians have been telling us to do for years— to eat a balanced diet. The problem is that in the United States we have had great trouble defining *what* a balanced diet is. Even more troublesome has been following through with dietary changes even when we know what they should be.

Fiber Intake

Average fiber intake in the United States is estimated at 15 to 20 gm/day. The sources of the fiber in our diet are

45 percent vegetables
35 percent cereals and legumes
20 percent fruits[1]

Some adults in rural Africa consume 130 gm of fiber daily by eating foods such as corn, millet, potatoes, and plantains. In the United States from 1909 to 1975, our intake of cereal fiber has *decreased* more than 50 percent.[2]

The National Cancer Institute (NCI) stated in 1984 that an optimum intake of fiber was about 25 to 35 gm/day. In 1986, NCI modified that recommendation, saying that Americans should try to double the amount of fiber they eat.[3] Some nutritionists believe we need as much as 30 gm of fiber for every 1,000 calories we eat.[4] An average man eating 2,000 calories would therefore need to eat 60 gm of fiber daily.

Frank's problem was that he increased his fiber intake too rapidly. He went from 14 to 42 gm/dl practically overnight. If you want to increase your fiber intake, do it gradually. Table 40 may help you in your planning. Remember, fiber exists only in plant foods. Meat, fish, and dairy products contain no fiber. That is why our usual diet of processed foods, meats, and dairy products has depleted our fiber intake to a dangerously low level, possibly causing the diseases discussed in the preceding chapter.

Using the information in table 40, you should be able to figure out how much fiber you are presently eating and how to gradually increase that amount over the next six months. Do not be discouraged if you find information elsewhere that contradicts the figures in table 40, for there *is* some variability. This table (from the American Dietetic Association) lists a medium-sized banana as having 2.4 gm of fiber, while the American Institute for Cancer Research lists the same size banana as having 4.0 gm.[5] The methods for analyzing dietary fiber have not yet been standardized. Even so, the reliable guides all tend to be similar enough to give excellent relative values for dietary fiber content.

Table 40

Dietary Fiber

Food	Serving size	Fiber per serving (gm)
BREAKFAST CEREALS		
All-Bran	⅓ cup (1 oz.)	8.5
100% Bran	½ cup (1 oz.)	8.4
Bran Buds	⅓ cup (1 oz.)	7.9
Corn Bran	⅔ cup (1 oz.)	5.4
Bran Chex	⅔ cup (1 oz.)	4.6
Cracklin' Bran	⅓ cup (1 oz.)	4.3
40% Bran	¾ cup (1 oz.)	4.0
Raisin Bran	¾ cup (1 oz.)	4.0
Most	⅔ cup (1 oz.)	3.5
Wheat germ	¼ cup (2 oz.)	3.4
Honey Bran	⅞ cup (1 oz.)	3.1
Shredded Wheat	⅔ cup (1 oz.)	2.6
Wheat 'n' Raisin Chex	¾ cup (1⅓ oz.)	2.5
Wheat Chex	⅔ cup (1⅓ oz.)	2.1
Frosted Mini Wheats	4 biscuits (1 oz.)	2.1
Wheaties	1 cup (1 oz.)	2.0
Total	1 cup (1 oz.)	2.0
Nutri-Grain, Wheat	¾ cup (1 oz.)	1.8
Nutri-Grain, Rye	¾ cup (1 oz.)	1.8
Nutri-Grain, Corn	¾ cup (1 oz.)	1.8
Nutri-Grain, Barley	¾ cup (1 oz.)	1.7
Graham Crackers	¾ cup (1 oz.)	1.7
Oatmeal, regular instant, cooked	¾ cup (1 oz.)	1.6
Grape-Nuts	¼ cup (1 oz.)	1.4
Heartland Natural Cereal	¼ cup (1 oz.)	1.3
Crispie Wheats n' Raisins	¾ cup (1 oz.)	1.3

Table 40 (continued)

Food	Serving size	Fiber per serving (gm)
BREAKFAST CEREALS (continued)		
Cheerios	1¼ cup (1 oz.)	1.1
100% Natural Cereal	¼ cup (1 oz.)	1.0
Sugar Smacks	¾ cup (1 oz.)	0.4
Corn Flakes	¼ cup (1 oz.)	0.3
Special K	1⅓ cup (1 oz.)	0.2
Rice Krispies	1 cup (1 oz.)	0.1
FRUITS		
Apple with skin	1 medium	3.5
Pear with skin	½ large	3.1
Raisins	¼ cup	3.1
Raspberries	½ cup	3.1
Prunes	3	3.0
Strawberries	1 cup	3.0
Apple without skin	1 medium	2.7
Orange	1	2.6
Pear without skin	½ large	2.5
Banana	1 medium	2.4
Blueberries	½ cup	2.0
Peach with skin	1	1.9
Dates	3	1.9
Apricot, fresh	3 medium	1.8
Grapefruit	½	1.6
Apricot, dried	5 halves	1.4
Peach without skin	1	1.2
Cherries, sweet	10	1.2
Cantaloupe	¼ melon	1.0
Pineapple	½ cup	1.1
Plums	5	0.9
Papaya juice	½ cup (4 oz.)	0.8
Grape juice	½ cup (4 oz.)	0.6

Table 40 (continued)

Food	Serving size	Fiber per serving (gm)
FRUITS (continued)		
Grapes	20	0.6
Grapefruit juice	½ cup (4 oz.)	0.5
Orange juice	½ cup (4 oz.)	0.4
Apple juice	½ cup (4 oz.)	0.4
Watermelon	1 cup	0.4
VEGETABLES, COOKED		
Peas	½ cup	3.6
Corn, canned	½ cup	2.9
Parsnips	½ cup	2.7
Potato with skin	1 medium	2.5
Carrots	½ cup	2.3
Brussels sprouts	½ cup	2.3
Broccoli	½ cup	2.2
Spinach	½ cup	2.1
Zucchini	½ cup	1.8
Sweet potatoes	½ medium	1.7
Turnips	½ cup	1.6
Beans, string, green	½ cup	1.6
Squash, summer	½ cup	1.4
Potato without skin	1 medium	1.4
Cabbage, white	½ cup	1.4
Cabbage, red	½ cup	1.4
Kale leaves	½ cup	1.4
Cauliflower	½ cup	1.1
Asparagus	½ cup	1.0
VEGETABLES, RAW		
Bean sprouts	½ cup	1.5
Tomato	1 medium	1.5
Spinach	1 cup	1.2

Table 40 (continued)

Food	Serving size	Fiber per serving (gm)
VEGETABLES, RAW (continued)		
Celery, diced	½ cup	1.1
Lettuce, sliced	1 cup	0.9
Mushrooms, sliced	½ cup	0.9
Onions, sliced	½ cup	0.8
Pepper, green, sliced	½ cup	0.5
Cucumbers	½ cup	0.4
LEGUMES		
Baked beans	½ cup	8.8
Kidney beans, cooked	½ cup	7.3
Navy beans, cooked	½ cup	6.0
Dried peas, cooked	½ cup	4.7
Lima beans, cooked	½ cup	4.5
Lentils, cooked	½ cup	3.7
BREADS, PASTAS, AND FLOURS		
Bran muffins	1	2.5
Crisp bread, rye	2 crackers	2.0
Crisp bread, wheat	2 crackers	1.8
Whole wheat bread	1 slice	1.4
Pumpernickel bread	1 slice	1.0
Cracked wheat bread	1 slice	1.0
Mixed grain bread	1 slice	0.9
French bread	1 slice	0.7
Raisin bread	1 slice	0.6
Bagels	1 bagel	0.6
Oatmeal bread	1 slice	0.5
White bread	1 slice	0.4
Pita bread (5 in.)	1 piece	0.4
Italian bread	1 slice	0.3
Spaghetti (whole wheat)	1 cup	3.9

Table 40 (continued)

Food	Serving size	Fiber per serving (gm)
BREADS, PASTAS, AND FLOURS (continued)		
Spaghetti (regular)	1 cup	1.1
Rice, brown	½ cup	1.0
Macaroni	1 cup	1.0
Rice, polished (white)	½ cup	0.2
GRAINS		
Bran, corn	1 oz.	17.6
Bran, wheat	1 oz.	11.7
Bran, oat	1 oz.	7.9
Wheatgerm	2 oz.	3.4
Rolled oats	1 oz.	1.6
NUTS		
Peanuts	10 nuts	1.4
Almonds	10 nuts	1.1
Filberts	10 nuts	0.8

Source: E. Lanza and R. Butrin, "Critical Review of Food Fiber Analysis and Data," Journal of the American Dietetic Association, 86 (June 1986): 737–39.

Adverse Effects

It is important to know that just because fiber is generally good for you, it is not *always* good for you. As Frank found out, too much fiber too fast can cause abdominal cramps, bloating, loose stools, and gas. Also, an increase in fiber intake can exacerbate certain diseases. These include acute or active inflammatory bowel disease (such as Crohn's disease and ulcerative colitis), acutely inflamed hemorrhoids, and inflamed "tics" (called diverticulitis).

Incidentally, the difference between diverticul*osis* (small balloon-like outpouchings of tissue in the colon) and divertic- ul*itis* is tremendous, similar to the difference between inac- tive or benign hemorrhoids and inflamed hemorrhoids. Think of a cyst on your arm, back, or ear that has been there for one or two years and has not bothered you at all. If the cyst becomes infected or inflamed, it swells and becomes irritated and quite painful. This analogy is similar to the situation when diver- ticula become inflamed (diverticulitis), the bowel becomes inflamed (colitis), or hemorrhoids become inflamed.

No one wants rough, heavy, bulky fiber passing over an irri- tated or inflamed area. That is why more fiber is exactly the *wrong* food to take when the body has one of the acute inflam- matory problems. Remember, though, that active inflamma- tion is quite unusual in these diseases; rather, these conditions are usually inactive, or in "remission." When this is the case, more fiber more often will benefit most people with an inflam- matory bowel problem, tics, or hemorrhoids.

Notes

1. S. Bingham and J. H. Cummings, *Medical Aspects of Dietary Fiber* (New York: Plenum Press, 1980), pp. 261–84.
2. S. Bingham, *Dietary Fiber, Fiber-Depleted Foods and Dis- ease* (London: Academic Press, 1985), pp. 94–96.
3. National Cancer Institute, U.S. Department of Health and Human Services, RHS, National Institutes of Health, *Diet, Nutrition, and Cancer Prevention: A Guide to Food Choices*, NIH publication no. 85-2711, November 1984; and *National Cancer Institute Statement: Diet and Cancer* (May 1986): 3.
4. L. Hachfeld, "Dietary Fiber in Perspective," unpublished report, 1984.
5. *Dietary Fiber to Lower Cancer Risk*, American Institute for Cancer Research, Information Series, September 1985.

Epilogue
Gaining Power by Eating Well

As you now know, the foods you eat and the liquids you drink can have a profound effect on you. They can influence how you feel, how you act, how often you are ill, your level of energy, what diseases you do or do not get, and even how and when you die.

Peter

I described 48-year-old Peter in chapter 1. He felt a great sense of power and self-confidence when he realized that he alone had been responsible for lowering his cholesterol level from 290 to 188 and his blood pressure from 149/90 to 126/84. He had literally changed his life (and death) around by using the power he had within him to eat and exercise in a more positive manner. Not only did Peter change his physical health, but he told me that he now felt more at peace emotionally and spiritually than he had in years.

Elizabeth

This 29-year-old woman was tormented for half of every month with mood swings, bloating, irritability, and sugar cravings. Birth control pills and diuretics had not helped control her premenstrual syndrome very much.

Elizabeth learned that by eating more whole grains, vegetables, and fruits plus markedly less sugar and salt, she could dramatically change how she felt in the two weeks before her menstrual periods. Actually making these changes mobilized her long-hidden sense of her own power and confidence and allowed her to begin to make substantial personal and career changes that were very beneficial to her.

This is not an uncommon pattern; I see it frequently in my practice. People such as Elizabeth are unable or unwilling to make the important decisions necessary for their lives to proceed. Instead, they decide to work on personal physical changes —for example, taking a more positive approach to eating. Such changes then improve not only the physical but also the emotional and spiritual aspects of their lives. The newfound sense of self-confidence and "I can do it" philosophy empower these individuals to move forward through life in a new, energetic, and confident manner.

Everybody

We can all empower ourselves by learning and taking a more positive approach to eating. Do not be concerned about what you might have to give up or avoid. Rather, focus on increasing the types of foods eaten by our ancestors for thousands of years: whole grains, vegetables, fruits, legumes, and water. Don't diet! Eat as much of these foods as you want. You won't gain weight, you will loose excess weight, and you won't feel deprived or starved. For an occasional reminder of the importance of your efforts, run your eye down the checklist in Table 41, which shows the symptoms and diseases related to common dietary culprits. Your new control over your diet will increase your chances of going through life with good health, more energy, and a sense of your own ability to truly affect how you feel and who you are!

Table 41

A Checklist of Symptoms and Diseases Associated with Common Dietary Culprits

	Caffeine	Salt	Sugar	Artificial Sweeteners	Fats	Milk	Processed Foods
Abdominal pains			X	X		X	
Acne					X	X	
Allergies			X	X	X	X	
Anal fissures							X
Anemia						X	
Angina	X				X	X	
Anorexia						X	
Anxiety	X		X				
Appendicitis							X
Appetite, loss of						X	
Arthritis					X		
Asthma						X	
Atherosclerosis					X	X	
Bed-wetting	X		X			X	
Behavior problems	X		X			X	
Birth defects	X			X			
Bloating		X			X	X	
Blood in stools						X	
Breast tenderness	X	X	X				
Bronchitis						X	
Cancer, certain types	X				X	X	X
Canker sores						X	
Chest pain					X		
Colic						X	
Colitis						X	X
Constipation		X			X	X	X
Coronary artery disease					X	X	

Table 41 (continued)

A Checklist of Symptoms and Diseases Associated with Common Dietary Culprits

	Caffeine	Salt	Sugar	Artificial Sweeteners	Fats	Milk	Processed Foods
Cramps, abdominal						X	X
Cravings for liquids		X					
Cravings for sweets			X	X			
Crohn's disease						X	X
Cystitis	X						
Dandruff						X	
Deafness					X		
Dental cavities			X			X	X
Depression	X		X	X		X	
Diabetes mellitus			X		X		X
Diarrhea	X			X		X	
Diverticulitis(osis)							X
Dizziness			X	X	X		
Ear infections (otitis)						X	
Eczema						X	
Edema		X					
Energy depletion						X	
Enuresis	X		X			X	
Excessive flus or colds			X				
Excessive sweating			X				
Fainting			X	X			
Fatigue	X	X	X		X	X	
Fibrocystic breasts	X						
Flatulence						X	
Frequent urination		X					
Gallbladder disease							X
Gas, intestinal				X		X	

Table 41 (continued)

A Checklist of Symptoms and Diseases Associated with Common Dietary Culprits

	Caffeine	Salt	Sugar	Artificial Sweeteners	Fats	Milk	Processed Foods
Gastritis	X					X	
Gout					X		
Gum disease (gingivitis)			X				
Headache	X	X	X	X		X	
Hearing loss					X		
Heartburn	X					X	
Heart disease (attack)	X		X		X	X	X
Heart palpitations	X		X				
Heart rate too fast	X		X				
Hemorrhoids		X					X
Hiatal hernia							X
High blood cholesterol	X		X			X	X
High blood pressure	X	X			X		
High blood triglycerides			X				X
Hives						X	
Hyperactivity	X		X			X	
Hypertension		X			X		X
Hypoglycemia	X		X				
Impotence					X		
Indigestion					X	X	
Inflammatory bowel disease						X	X
Insomnia	X					X	
Intermittent claudication (circulation-related leg cramps)					X		

Table 41 (continued)

A Checklist of Symptoms and Diseases Associated with Common Dietary Culprits

	Caffeine	Salt	Sugar	Artificial Sweeteners	Fats	Milk	Processed Foods
Irritability			X			X	
Irritable colon			X	X		X	X
Irritation of lips, mouth, or tongue						X	
Itching			X	X		X	
Itchy anus	X		X			X	
Joint aches			X			X	
Kidney stones			X		X		
Leg pains			X		X		
Lethargy	X	X	X			X	X
Memory loss			X	X			
Menopause, too late					X		
Menstrual cramps				X	X		
Menstruation onset, too early					X		
Moodiness, mood swings			X	X			
Multiple sclerosis						X	
Muscle aches			X			X	
Nausea				X		X	
Nephritis					X		
Nightmares	X						
Obesity			X		X		X
Osteoporosis	X		X		X		
Panic disorders	X						
Peripheral vascular disease					X		
Phlegm and mucus, excess						X	

Table 41 (continued)

A Checklist of Symptoms and Diseases Associated with Common Dietary Culprits

	Caffeine	Salt	Sugar	Artificial Sweeteners	Fats	Milk	Processed Foods
Pneumonia (recurrent)						X	
Polyps, colon							X
Polysystemic chronic candidiasis			X				
Poor concentration			X				
Postnasal drip						X	
Premenstrual syndrome	X	X	X		X		
Prostatitis	X						
Protein in urine						X	
Puffy feet and ankles		X					
Pulmonary embolus							X
Rectal pain	X						
Restlessness	X		X			X	
Ringing in the ears	X	X					
Seizures					X		
Senility					X		
Sinusitis						X	
Skin nodules					X		
Skin rashes			X	X	X		
Spastic colon			X	X		X	X
Strep throat (recurrent)						X	
Stroke					X		
Stuffy nose						X	
Swollen voice box					X		

Table 41 (continued)

A Checklist of Symptoms and Diseases Associated
with Common Dietary Culprits

	Caffeine	Salt	Sugar	Artificial Sweeteners	Fats	Milk	Processed Foods
Throat lump (globus)	X						
Thrombophlebitis							X
Tonsillitis (recurrent)						X	
Transient ischemic attack					X		
Tremors	X		X				
Ulcerative colitis						X	X
Ulcers	X					X	
Urethritis	X						
Urine frequency	X						
Vaginal discharge			X				
Vaginal itching			X				
Vaginitis			X				
Varicose veins							X
Vertigo			X	X	X		
Vomiting						X	
Weakness		X	X				
Yeast infection			X				

A Final Note

Eat for Health does not cover all the side effects of all the foods we eat or drink. For example, for the sake of brevity, I did not discuss the well-documented problems and diseases related to alcohol consumption. These include liver disease, gastritis, ulcers, esophagitis, oral and other cancers, pancreatitis, automobile and other accidents, relationship problems, plus many others. Other important sources of problems from foods not covered in this book (or mentioned only briefly) are these:

- food additives
- pesticides
- animal drugs
- pollutants
- toxic molds

Most people do not realize that more than 90 percent of the *additives* in food are two of the food types we have already examined: sugar and salt. The other 3,000 additives include dyes (such as Red Number 3), flavorings (such as monosodium glutamate [MSG]), preservatives (BHT, BHA), curing agents for meat (nitrites, nitrates), and multiple others. Some of these additives have been suspected of causing cancer. MSG can cause the allergic reaction called the "Chinese Restaurant Syndrome." Dr. Benjamin Feingold and others have shown that artificial colors and flavors plus foods containing salicylates (salts of salicylic acid used as preservatives) cause hyperactivity (attention-deficit disorders) in some children. Other studies, however, contradict Dr. Feingold's findings. I believe a small number of hyperactivity problems are caused by these food additives.

Some *pesticides*, such as DDT, have been implicated as causing cancer. Another pesticide, called parathion, can cause interference with nervous system enzymes. Still others are suspected of reducing male sperm counts, thereby leading to infertility.

Drugs used in animals received lots of publicity in the 1970s. It was discovered then that DES (diethylstilbestrol), a hormone used as a growth stimulant in cattle, caused cancer. This same drug, as mentioned earlier, was used in the 1940s in pregnant women in an attempt to prevent miscarriages. Unfortunately, it was found to cause cancer of the vagina and cervix in some of the users' daughters and occasional testicle cancers in their sons.

Other drugs used in animals, such as antibiotics, can remain as a residue in small amounts in meat and milk. For susceptible individuals such as Gary, discussed in part V, allergic reactions can result from ingesting such animal products. Gary's persistent rash was found to be caused by penicillin present in the milk he drank.

Pollutants are primarily of two types:

- chlorinated hydrocarbons (PCBs, dioxins)
- heavy metals (lead, mercury, cadmium)

PCBs are suspected of having caused acne, birth defects, cancer, decreased immunity, and liver disease. Dioxins may cause acne, cirrhosis of the liver, kidney problems, mental disturbances such as depression and poor memory, and ulcers.

Health problems relating to an accumulation of heavy metals cover the entire spectrum of symptoms and diseases. These include abdominal pains, heart disease, high blood pressure, and muscle weakness. Lead can sneak into our bodies when we eat canned foods, since tin cans are seamed with leaded solder. Another source of lead is the calcium-containing supplement in some bonemeal tablets. Mercury can be found in some fish, and cadmium can wash off rusted water pipes and into our drinking water.

An example of a *toxic mold* that we might ingest is aflatoxin. Many foods can be contaminated with this mold poison, but peanuts (and, therefore, peanut butter) are especially vulnerable. Aflatoxin is one of the world's most potent promoters of liver cancer in animals.

These few examples suggest why another book could be written about the common diseases and problems caused by foods and liquids not even covered in *Eat for Health*. It is important to remember that you can avoid most additives by eating a diet composed primarily of whole grains, fruits, vegetables, and legumes.

As I mentioned with regard to the foods themselves, I would appreciate hearing from people who have reduced their own symptoms and controlled or eliminated diseases by avoiding additives, pesticides, animal drugs, pollutants, or toxic molds.

Enjoy your food — and your good health! Feel a new sense of power in your ability to track down and solve some of the nagging problems that may have been bothering you for years. Congratulate yourself for taking the initial steps in eating both for pleasure and physical well-being.

Helpful Books for Healthy Eating

1. John A. McDougall, M.D., and Mary A. McDougall. *The McDougall Plan*. New Jersey: New Century Publishers, 1983.

2. Aveline Kushi. *Macrobiotic Cooking*. New York: Warner Books, 1985.

3. Jane Brody. *Jane Brody's Good Food Book*. New York: Norton, 1985.

4. Laurel Robertson, Carol Flinders, and Bronwen Godfrey. *Laurel's Kitchen*. Petaluma, Calif.: Nilgiri Press, 1976.

5. Laurel Robertson, Carol Flinders, and Brian Ruppenthal. *The New Laurel's Kitchen*. Berkeley, Calif.: Ten Speed Press, 1986.

6. Francis Moore Lappé. *Diet for a Small Planet, Tenth Anniversary Edition*. New York: Ballantine, 1982.

7. C. Norman Shealy, M.D., Ph.D. *Speedy Gourmet: A Wholesome Alternative to Fast Foods*. Fair Grove, Mo.: Brindabella Books, 1984.

8. Mollie Katzen. Moosewood Cookbook Series: Berkeley, Calif.: Ten Speed Press.
   The Moosewood Cookbook, 1977.
   The Enchanted Broccoli Forest, 1982.
   New Recipes From Moosewood Restaurant, 1987.

9. Mankato Heart Health Program. *Cooking á La Heart*. Mankato, Minn.: Mankato Heart Health Program, 1988.

Index

References to figures and tables are printed in boldface type.

and, 59, 99, 106; dairy products
and, 143, 145, 146, 173; fats in
diet and, 109, 120; fiber and,
197, 207; processed foods and,
190; sodium and, 37, 41; sugar
and, 59, 106. *See also* Edema;
Premenstrual syndrome.
Blood cholesterol levels. *See*
Cholesterol, levels in blood of.
Blood clots. *See* Pulmonary
Embolus; Thrombophlebitis.
Blood pressure: caffeine and, 7,
19, 22; fats in diet and, 109,
111, 112, 118, 127, 141; high, 7,
22, 37, 38, 39, 65, 109, 118,
127, 218; processed foods and,
177, 194–95; safe range for, 19,
38, 112; sodium and, 37, 38,
39, 52; sugar and, 79
Blood sugar. *See* Diabetes;
Hypoglycemia.
Body fat. *See* Fat, body.
Bologna, 131, **132, 139**
Bone fractures and disorders,
calcium intake and, 160–67,
162, 163
Bones, thinning of. *See*
Osteoporosis.
Books. *See* Reading, recommended.
Bouillon, 32
Bowel disorders. *See* Colon and
bowel, disorders of.
Brain. *See* Central nervous sys-
tem; Strokes.
Brainard, J. B., 41–42
Bran, 19, 187, 201, **207**
Bread, **4;** calcium in, **165;** dairy-
free, **175;** fats in, **133, 134;**
fiber in, **198–200, 206–7;**
sodium in, 44, **45, 49;** white
vs. whole wheat, 178–79, **179,**
180; whole wheat, 61, 97
Breakfast, 44, **45,** 60, 61, 74, 131;
198. *See also specific foods.*
Breast milk: cow's milk vs., 153,

160, 164, 171–72. *See also*
Nursing mothers.
Breasts: caffeine and, 7, 15–16,
18–19; cancer of, 15–16, 18–19,
109, 113, 115, 117; **122, 123,**
124–25, **124,** 187; cysts and
lumps in, 15, 16; fats in diet
and, 109, 113, 117, **122, 123,**
124–25, **124;** fibrocystic disease of, 7, 15–16; sodium and,
37, 42, 52; sugar and, 59; tenderness of, 7, 37, 42, 52, 59, 68
Breath, shortness of: sodium
and, 38
Broccoli, **165, 205**
Bronchitis. *See* Respiratory
problems.
Broth, 32–33
Brown sugar, 84, **85**
Burkitt, D. P., 189
Butter, **135**
Buttermilk, **133, 166**

Cabbage, **133, 166**
Cacao seeds, 8
Cadmium, in foods, 218
Caffeine: addiction to, 8, 10,
14–15, 17–18, 31, 77; adverse
effects of, 1, 2, 3, 5, 8–25, 36,
41, 42, 161, 164, 166; alternatives to, 32–36; beneficial
effects of, 8–9; elimination
diet and, 10, 11, 12, 13, 15, 16,
19–20, 21–22, 24, 25, 31–32,
33; lowering intake of, 27–36;
safe quantities of, 19, 22, 23,
36; sources of, 8, **28;** withdrawal from, 14–15, 31–32. *See
also* Caffeine content;
Decaffeination; *specific body
parts, diseases, and symptoms;
specific foods and drinks.*
Caffeine content: of chocolate
and cocoa, 20, **28;** of coffee, 21,
22, **28;** of various foods and

Books That Transform Lives

WAY OF THE PEACEFUL WARRIOR
by Dan Millman
*"It may even change the lives of many . . .
who peruse its pages."*—DR. STANLEY KRIPPNER

**OPENING TO CHANNEL:
HOW TO CONNECT WITH YOUR GUIDE**
by Sanaya Roman and Duane Packer, Ph.D.
*This breakthrough book is the first
step-by-step guide to the art of channeling.*

TALKING WITH NATURE
by Michael J. Roads
*"From Australia comes a major new writer . . .
a magnificent book!"*—RICHARD BACH

CREATING MONEY
by Sanaya Roman and Duane Packer, Ph.D.
The bestselling authors of OPENING TO CHANNEL
offer the reader the keys to abundance.

SEEDS OF LIGHT
by Peter Rengel
*". . . contains a widely varied collection
of pearls of poetic wisdom."*—PROMETHEAN NETWORK

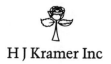

H J Kramer Inc

Books That Transform Lives

THE EARTH LIFE SERIES
by Sanaya Roman, Channel for Orin

LIVING WITH JOY, BOOK I
"I like this book because it describes the way I feel about so many things."—VIRGINIA SATIR

PERSONAL POWER
THROUGH AWARENESS, BOOK II
"Every sentence contains a pearl. . . ."—LILIAS FOLAN

JOY IN A WOOLLY COAT
by Julie Adams Church
Destined to become a classic, JOY IN A WOOLLY COAT *is about living with, loving, and letting go of treasured animal friends.*

SINGING MAN
by Neil Anderson
"One of the finest allegories of our time . . . a story of everyman in transition."—JEAN HOUSTON

WAY OF THE PEACEFUL WARRIOR
An Audio Cassette
Read by Author Dan Millman
A 96-minute abridged version of the metaphysical classic, WAY OF THE PEACEFUL WARRIOR.

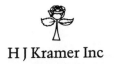

H J Kramer Inc